A Gaia **Busy Person's** Guide

Massage

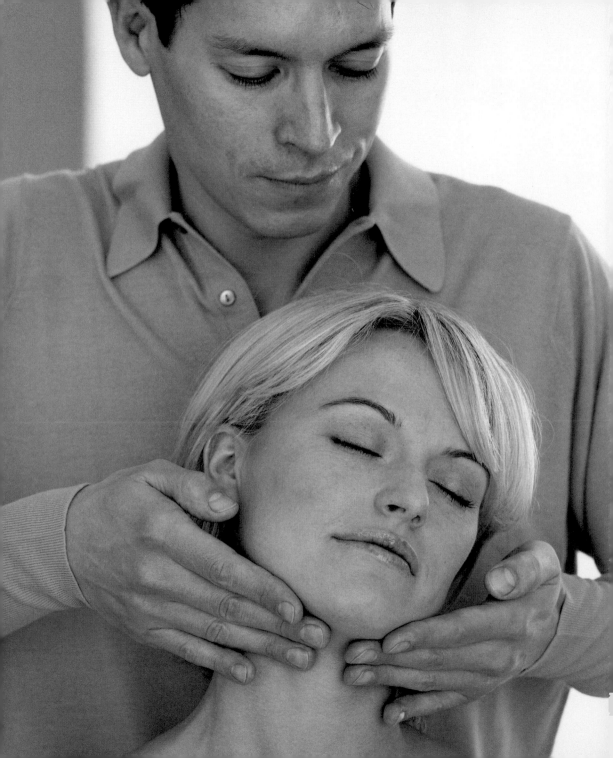

A Gaia **Busy Person's** Guide

Massage

Soothe away the tensions and anxieties of a busy lifestyle

Eilean Bentley

Gaia Books

A Gaia Original

Books from Gaia celebrate the vision of Gaia, the self-sustaining living Earth, and seek to help its readers live in greater personal and planetary harmony.

Direction Lyn Hemming, Patrick Nugent
Production Jim Pope, Louise Hall
Editor Fiona Biggs, Kelly Thompson
Design Phil Gamble
Photography Ruth Jenkinson

GAIA

® This is a Registered Trade Mark of Gaia Books
an imprint of Octopus Publishing Group, 2–4 Heron Quays, London,
E14 4JP

ISBN 1 85675 249 6
EAN 9 781856 752497

A catalogue record of this book is available from the British Library.

Printed and bound in China by Toppan

10 9 8 7 6 5 4 3 2 1

Contents

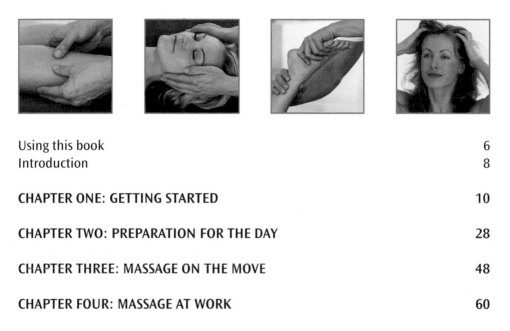

Using this book

This book offers a selection of massage techniques drawn from Shiatsu, head massage, acupressure, aromatherapy, therapeutic massage, meditation, and the use of crystals in re-balancing energy, to take you through busy days and into relaxing evenings. You can use it to guide you into a daily calming routine that will help to energize and revitalize your life, or you can dip into it to discover quick ways to defuse a tense situation, to overcome afternoon tiredness, or to help alleviate the daily aches and pains that can adversely affect your performance.

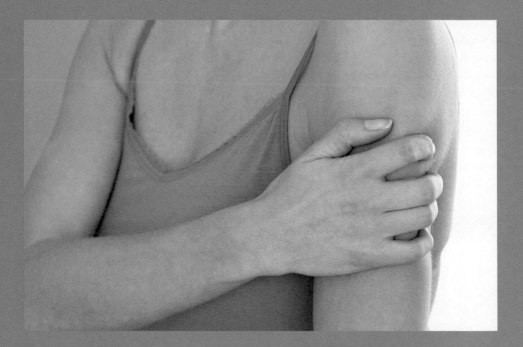

Basic techniques are explained in Chapter One. You will learn how to use your hands, your arms, and even your feet to bring good health and well-being to you and your partner. You are also introduced to different therapies and exercises and the role of crystals in helping to maintain a good balance of energy.

Chapter Two takes you through a daily routine that will help to get you started for the busy day. This covers breathing and exercises to wake up every cell in your body. It also includes self-help routines for some of the more common ailments that can strike because of stress, the daily use of computers, difficulties at work, and the build-up of tensions during the average day. It ends with a chakra meditation, which, if practised regularly, will transform your life by re-charging your body's energy centres, removing any sense of lack in your life, improving your creativity and awareness, and calming your mind and body.

Chapters Three and Four deal with your daily working life, from travelling to work, through various times where you can take short re-energizing massage breaks, to the later part of the day when you may need some real help with headache, tiredness, and lack of concentration.

Chapter Five takes you into the evening at home, where you and your partner can start the process of relaxation by giving each other a head massage.

Chapter Six provides the techniques for a long, relaxing full body massage session that will totally de-stress and relax you both, ready for the next day.

THE POWER OF TOUCH
Good diet, regular exercise, and massage are well-established ways of boosting the body's own healing powers, energy, and resistance to disease. Even if you do become ill, regular massage will speed recovery.

Introduction

The healing, communicative, and bonding power of touch has been very well understood down through the centuries. All cultures, civilizations, and communities, human or animal, have used touch as a means of communication and bringing their society together.

Touch is not only a comforting and pleasurable means of relaxing; it is also a very necessary part of being alive. Research with institutionalized orphans has shown that denying touch is very detrimental to the basic health of the child. Those who were touched, even if they had succumbed to serious illness, were brought back to and maintained good health. Other studies included those undergoing major surgery and suffering life-threatening and long-term illness. In each case, including massage in their treatment resulted in faster, less painful, and longer-lasting recovery.

WHAT IS MASSAGE?

From the desire to touch and be touched sprang many, varied therapies. Some use only the simplest touch of holding a hand and wishing, or channelling, good health and well-being to the one being treated.

Others are elaborate, energetic, even gymnastic in their approach. However, as the great Shiatsu master Shizuto Masunaga has said, "When you begin, you give long technical treatments. When you get better, your treatments get shorter." So, a few well-spent moments of treatment done with care and good intention can bring just as many benefits as a long routine executed with precision.

So what exactly is massage? It has been described as the restoration and maintenance of good health by means of manipulation of the body's soft tissue. That's the short answer. Massage is also a holistic therapy, which considers the whole person, their choices of food, drink, occupation, and pastimes. With a wide variety of disciplines from which to choose, there is treatment or therapy to suit every person or problem.

HOW IT WORKS

Some massage therapies work on muscles, joints, ligaments, and tendons. They work firmly to move tissue over tissue, so ridding the body of the toxic build-up that can cause physical problems such as arthritis, rheumatism, and sciatica. Others work in a more gentle way, reaching far within the body's energy systems to release deep-rooted problems. Even entrenched emotional problems can be moved and cleared out of your body and mind by sensitive massage.

Is it dangerous? Messing about with your mind as well as your body may sound frightening. Many people will run from exposing their innermost feelings. Even though you may sometimes feel a little emotionally wobbly after a massage you will always be in control of yourself. This is a normal reaction and it will clear up after a few days. You may even find that deep-rooted problems will surface and clear and this will cause you to feel much more alive and free.

LEARNING THE TECHNIQUES

To enable you to treat specific ailments or problems you should undertake a professional training course in whichever therapy you choose to study. However, to give a massage that will very effectively release everyday problems that have no medical cause, you don't need any professional training. Working gently, with loving care, while wishing good health and well-being to yourself or the person you are working on will prepare you to meet life's next challenge.

TAKING CARE OF YOURSELF

If you are going to look after the health and well-being of others you must first look after yourself. It is very important to constantly refresh your own levels of energy to avoid becoming worn-out, depleted, or ill. Regular practice of breathing, meditation, and bodywork such as arm swinging will help you to develop your basic fitness, awareness, ability to focus and concentrate, stamina, flexibility, and reflexes. Even if you are only working on yourself, regular practice of the exercises will improve your techniques and deepen the effectiveness of the massage.

Eileen Bentley

CHAPTER ONE

Getting started

Massage needs no special equipment. You don't even need to use your hands. Many therapists use only their feet and knees. And you don't need to take your clothes off. In fact, for many massage therapies it is better to wear light clothing to provide a barrier between the giver and the receiver, since the touch of bare skin can distract the giver from a full awareness of the body's energy.

Regular massage can relieve stress, tension, tiredness, aching joints, headaches, insomnia, digestive problems, and emotionally related disturbances such as Crohn's disease, irritable bowel syndrome (IBS), and asthma. Massage is relaxing, pleasurable, bonding, and regenerating. It can help you to clear your thoughts, increase your creativity, open your awareness, lose weight, release depression, strengthen joints, loosen muscles, stretch tendons, increase overall flexibility, and much more. The healing power of massage is greatly enhanced by combining it with meditation and visualization, encouraging the receiver's own healing intentions to support the giver. Using essential oils and crystals can increase the potency of the treatment.

When you arrive at work, mentally build into your day at least one 30-minute break where you can give yourself a revitalizing workout with head massage, loosening exercises, and calming breathing exercises.

If you find yourself daydreaming it means that you need a break to gather your thoughts. Turn your daydreams into short meditations and take a few moments to massage your neck or shoulders. Try to get away from your phones and computer for 15 minutes to recharge your batteries. Take another quick refresher at the close of the day, before you set off for home. It will calm you before you have to tackle rush-hour chaos. Have a good, relaxing massage at least twice a week to regenerate your whole being.

Techniques

Here are a few basic techniques to get you started. Once you have mastered the general principles you may find that you start making up your own strokes and sequences. Go with what feels good for you and your partner. Don't worry too much about the right way or the wrong way, just go.

■ *Stroking* Use flat hands, fingers, thumbs, even your forearms, in a smooth, flowing action, running lightly over the body in straight lines, circles, or long sweeps. You can use both hands together, covering a large area such as the back, or one hand after the other, giving a continuous flow of following strokes. Place your hands (or fingers, thumbs, or forearms) on the area being worked and glide lightly over the surface, in your chosen direction.

■ *Rotations* Using firm pressure, work your fingers, thumbs, or elbows in small circles over one spot.

■ *Kneading* Good for large muscles over the shoulders and back, but can be used in other areas if you moderate the pressure. Use your fist or the heel of your hand against the pressure of your other palm, thumbs working against fingers, or fingers against thumbs, in a pinching action that works a large area.

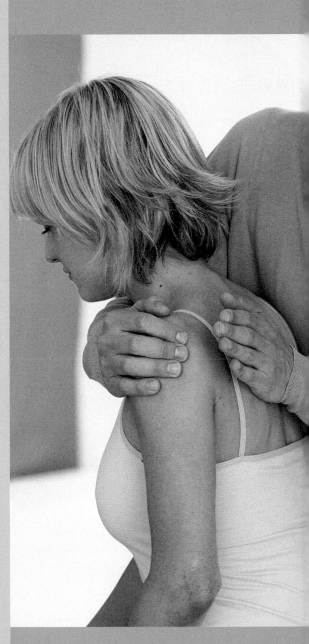

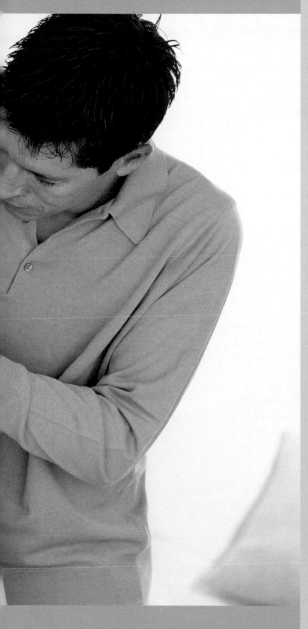

The pressure should be firm but never to the point of pain.

■ *Pinching* Similar to kneading, but you pick up small areas of flesh between your fingers and thumbs. Again, be firm without causing any actual pain.

■ *Wringing* Taking the muscle between both hands, twist your hands in opposite directions. This is just like wringing out wet towels. It should work the muscle fibres together without pain.

■ *Pressure* Use your fingers, thumbs, fists, elbows, feet, knees, or any part of your body that can exert a still, steady pressure on the relevant area to master this energy-toning technique.

■ *Hacking/tapping/pummelling* You can use the sides of your hands or the backs of your hands (hacking), your fingertips (tapping), your fist, or clasped hands (pummelling). This is a rapid drumming movement, using one hand after the other, or, in the case of your clasped hands, both hands together. The pressure varies from light tapping to heavy pummelling, with hacking coming somewhere in between.

■ *Knuckling* Usually you use the large knuckles of your fingers, but you can also use the smaller knuckles to work more delicate areas, such as the face.

Different types of massage

The techniques in this book have been drawn from a variety of massages. This is not a comprehensive study of each massage, more a selection of moves, pressure points, and steps, which can be quickly and easily used by any beginner.

SHIATSU (01)

This is a slow, gentle, relaxing form of massage. All that may seem to be going on is someone leaning with their fingers, thumbs, or arms on another person or gently wringing their limbs. However, the power of Shiatsu is deep. Positive intention is all-important – this is how the practitioner controls the direction and strength of the energy passing through the recipient. Working on tsubos (vital Japanese pressure points) while focusing on the inner energy channels (meridians) of the receiver, the giver slowly releases unhealthy blockages and rebalances the flow of energy within the body.

HEAD MASSAGE (02)

Massaging your head, neck, and shoulders releases tension in the muscles of the upper body, relieving headaches, destressing your mind and body, and moving toxins out of your system. Working the tsubos on the many meridians within this area can improve the health of the internal organs, and tone and refresh your whole being.

AROMATHERAPY

For many centuries healers have used the essences of plants to assist in the curing of many ailments. Aromatherapy is a very relaxing, pleasurable way of absorbing those powerful, healing oils into our bodies. There is an oil for almost every problem, and combining oils with the power of touch results in a therapy that is one of the most relaxing, calming, and refreshing ways to unwind after a busy day.

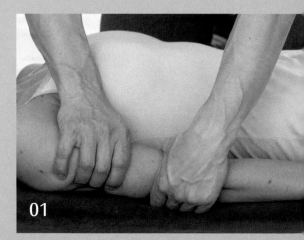

01

ACUPRESSURE (03)

Unlike Shiatsu, which works on meridians and pressure points that are not necessarily in fixed positions, acupressure and acupuncture both use fixed points. They can be activated by a firm touch, a needle (in the case of acupuncture), or an electrical current. The pressure points are very responsive and can relieve pain, sickness, and stiffness in muscles and joints very quickly and effectively. To get the best from an acupressure treatment you must apply firm pressure for at least a minute to each point used.

THERAPEUTIC MASSAGE

For deep muscle, joint, and other problems, the strong manipulative techniques of therapeutic massage can bring great relief. The intention of the giver is fixed on the structure of your body, so that they are aware of underlying problems within muscles, organs, and the skeletal, digestive, circulatory, and nervous systems. The healing work relies on the movement of tissue over tissue, which releases toxic waste build-up from your muscles and joints. Therapeutic massage, with its medical origins, is more clinical than the more ancient and traditional systems of Shiatsu and acupressure.

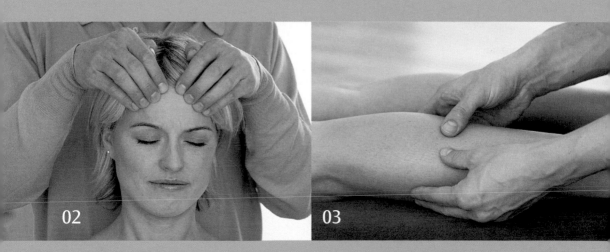

02

03

Pressure points for massage

Acupressure points are not magic buttons that can turn health problems off like a light switch. But used regularly and with care, they can rebalance the health of your body and mind so that the problems become less frequent in occurrence and intensity.

Having said that, sometimes the points can work swiftly and effectively to ease a problem. I have treated people with back pain, headaches, tension-related sickness, and breathing and mobility problems, whose symptoms have apparently cleared up immediately. However, in many cases, it has been a first aid treatment – it alleviated symptoms, but didn't deal with the underlying problem, which required care and further treatment.

The danger with "push-button" cures is that you will overstrain your system by returning too quickly to your old ways, and the problem that prompted you to seek treatment will return. Pain and sickness are often lifestyle problems. The acupressure points here can help only as an addition to good posture, healthy eating, good sleep, relaxed mind, and positive mental habits and practices.

FOR THE TOP OF THE HEAD AND THE BACK OF THE BODY

- *GV20* Poor memory and concentration, headaches, mild depression. Clears the brain and calms the mind.
- *GV16* Colds, headaches, sore throats, nosebleeds.
- *GB20* Stiff neck, tension headaches, insomnia, hypertension. Use with GV16 to help relieve the symptoms of colds.
- *B10* Stress, tension, anxiety, insomnia. Opens the awareness, calms the mind, relaxes the body, relieves colds and flu.
- *GB21* Tension and tiredness in the shoulders and neck, frozen shoulder. Relaxes the mind, reduces nervous stress, anger, irritability. Very energizing.
- *B13* Breathing difficulties, detoxifying.
- *B23, B47* Relieve lower backache, rebalance energy in the kidneys and digestive system.
- *TH4* Soothes wrist pain.
- *LI4* Headaches, mild depression, general pain. Anaesthetic and detoxifying.
- *K3* Water retention, swollen feet, sleeping difficulties. Protects the immune system. Very useful and safe in pregnancy, eases labour.
- *B60* Lower back pain, joint and rheumatic pain in the lower body.

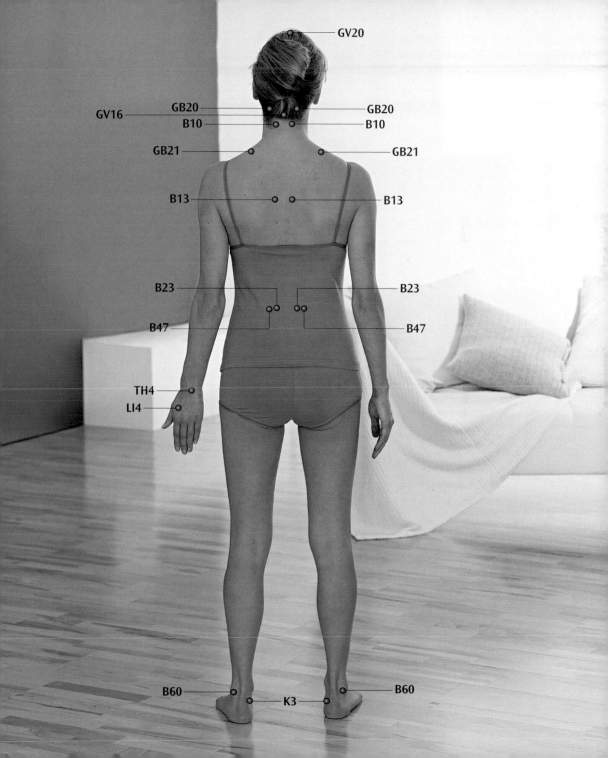

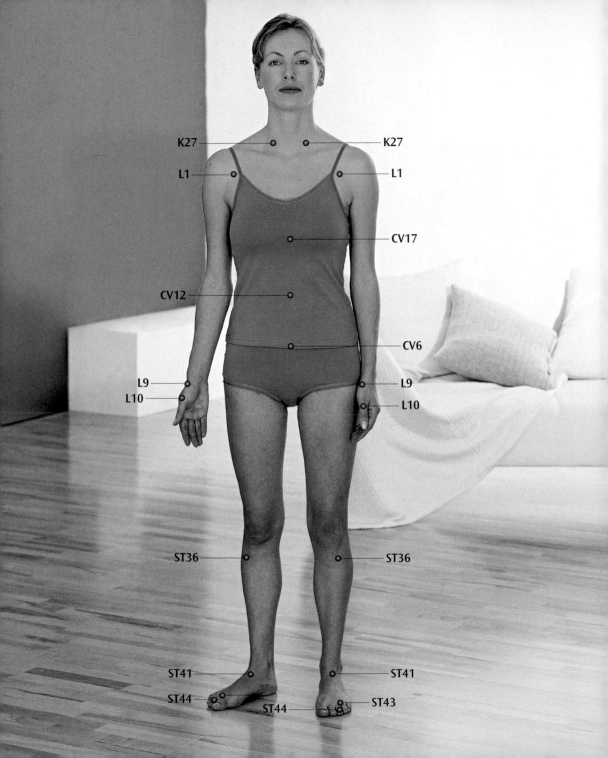

FOR THE FACE AND THE FRONT OF THE BODY

- **GV25** Depression, weak immune system. Clears the mind, calms fears, relaxes the body.
- **B2, GV24.5** Eye and sinus problems, headaches, and other facial pain.
- **B1** Nosebleeds, tired and aching eyes.
- **LI20** Head colds, nasal congestion.
- **ST2** Good for the complexion, relieves eye strain.
- **ST3** Sinuses, tired, dry eyes.
- **GV26** Dizziness, fainting, cramp.
- **K27** Sore throat, coughing, hiccups, anxiety. Rebalances the kidneys.
- **L1** Asthma, breathing difficulties. Stabilizes the emotions, eases confusion, clears the mind.

- **CV17** Mild depression, grief.
- **CV12** Emotional problems, stress, digestive problems.
- **CV6** Trapped wind, constipation, lower back problems. Revitalizes the body's energy flow.
- **L9** Relieves asthma, bronchitis. Reduces fear, anger, anxiety.
- **L10** Lung congestion, emotional upset, wrist pain.
- **ST36** Sickness, nausea. Balances the digestive system, stimulates the immune system, boosts energy.
- **ST41** Fear, nervous tension. Ankle and heel pain.
- **ST43, ST44** Excess wind, sickness and nausea, facial pain, nosebleeds, aching teeth and gums.

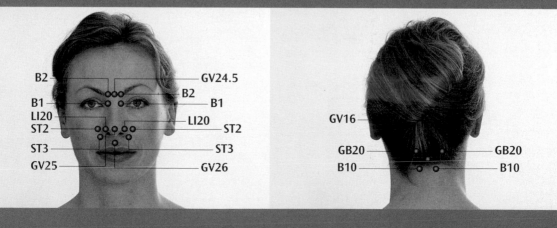

Aromatherapy massage

An aromatherapy massage, either as a self-treatment or working with a partner, is a simple, extremely effective way to unwind at the end of a day. The techniques are very safe and easy to use. They are mainly long, smooth, stroking movements, done with the flat palms, fingers, thumbs, and sometimes the forearms, working on bare skin. This technique combines the senses of touch and smell to give a relaxing, calming treatment.

You don't need a special working surface such as a couch – you can work on the floor on folded blankets covered by a sheet. This allows you to use your body weight to increase the strength of the stroke but still gives the feeling of rhythmic effortlessness.

CAUTION
■ *Do not use oil on the eyes as this may irritate the delicate tissues.*
■ *Do not exert strong pressure on the soft tissue of the abdomen.*

OILS

Always dilute essential oils in a carrier oil (grapeseed, sunflower, sweet almond, sesame, soya) for massage. The usual proportions are 15 drops of essential oil to 60ml of carrier oil for a full-body massage. For a smaller area such as the face use 5 drops to 30ml.

■ *Angelica* Calming, good for digestion, antiseptic, antiviral. Do not use during pregnancy. Photo-toxic, so avoid exposure to sunlight after use.

■ *Chamomile* Relaxing, anti-inflammatory.

■ *Citronella* Good for aches and pains. Also good as an insect repellent. Do not use this oil during pregnancy.

■ *Clary sage* Warming and soothing. Do not use this oil during pregnancy.

■ *Eucalyptus* Antiseptic, decongestant, antiviral.

■ *Frankincense* Warming, relaxing, uplifting.

■ *Geranium* Soothing, relaxing, antidepressant.

■ *Jasmine* Uplifting, relaxing, good for cramp.

■ *Lavender* Soothing, relaxing, antiseptic.

■ *Lemon* Refreshing, stimulating, antiseptic. Photo-toxic, so avoid exposure to sunlight after use.

■ *Myrrh* Warming, relaxing, anti-inflammatory. Do not use this oil during pregnancy.

■ *Peppermint* Cooling, good for digestion, mentally stimulating. Never use undiluted or before sleeping.

■ *Petitgrain* Soothing, calming, antidepressant.

■ *Rosemary* Stimulating, refreshing. Do not use this oil during pregnancy or if you suffer from epilepsy.

■ *Tea tree* Antifungal, antiseptic.

■ *Ylang-ylang* Euphoric, aphrodisiac, relaxing. Use in moderation.

Aromatherapy: basic strokes

STROKING (01)

You can use strong pressure on the back of the body –
for the legs use your palms, fingers, and fists; for the
back you can also use your forearms. You can use both
hands together or one hand after the other, keeping
up a continuous rhythm. Work from feet to knees,
repeating the stroke three or four times. Then work
from knees to buttocks in the same way, then up over
the back and up the backs of the arms. You can also
work in the opposite direction, starting at the
shoulders, moving down the arms, the back, and,
finally, the legs. Work systematically and rhythmically.

When stroking the front of the body, start at the
shoulders and work down the arms, then down the
front of the chest to the abdomen. You can use a
stronger pressure over the front of the legs, down to
the feet. Use a firm stroke on the feet as a light touch
can tickle and this is not relaxing.

When massaging yourself or a partner, use only
your fingers on the face, moving in a light upward
direction. Starting under the chin, stroke up to the
temples three or four times, then across the lips and
under the nose, across the nose to the temple area,
and across the forehead from the centre to the sides.

RAKING

Using the pads of your fingertips rake upward over the
legs and arms. Rake over the back from side to spine,
one side at a time. Use firm but not hard pressure,
and the lightest pressure over the face.

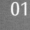

THUMB ROTATIONS AND PRESSURE (02)

For rotations, move your thumb(s) in small circles to work firmly into the area. For pressure, drop your weight on to your thumbs and hold for a few moments. With a lighter hold, you can also use rotations and pressure over the neck and facial area.

KNEADING (03)

For strongly muscled areas, support your partner's body with one hand and, using firm pressure with the fist of your other hand, slide your fist over the body toward your supporting hand. On all other areas use your thumbs, sliding in a firm pressure toward your outstretched fingers in a pinching action.

FRICTION RUB

Rub the palms or edges of your hands over your partner's body with an alternate sawing action, one hand after the other.

PUMMELLING/HACKING

The strongest action is with two hands clasped together and used to pound the flesh. Using your hands individually, one after the other, will give a rapid drumming treatment. Cupped hands or fingers are the lightest and are most suitable for more sensitive areas.

Crystals and massage

Many therapists are achieving very good results by giving their clients crystals to hold during treatment. The crystals seem to deepen the treatment and relax and clear not only the person being treated, but also the person giving the treatment. After all, our bodies and minds are crystals in solution. Even the solid matter of tissue forms crystals if it is dried, and our spirit is pure energy.

Crystals are also very beneficial for the energy of the room in which they are placed. All stones work at their best when they are in the environment in which they were formed. Their energies are complemented fully by all that is around them. They are at home. However, it is not usually practical for many people to go to the home of a crystal. The crystals must travel to you. During that journey they can pick up many energies, from the person who mined or found them, right through the many transactions that eventually brought them to you. Neutralizing these energies is a necessary process through which they must go if you are to be able to access their properties free from any other influence.

There are many ways of doing this. You can run them under cold water to earth the energy. If you have a collection of crystals you can cleanse any new ones by surrounding them with your existing collection. You can also cleanse them by placing your energy within them. Hold the stone in your hand and visualize your hands filling with light. See the crystal absorbing the light and releasing any negativity. Earth this negativity by visualizing it flowing down into the ground. This is a good method to use if you are going to programme the stones for a specific purpose, such as healing. The way I prefer is to wrap the stones in a natural material, such as cotton, and bury them in the garden for a few days. This has the advantage of balancing their energies with those of the land about them. It gives them a new home.

The relationship between a crystal and its holder is very like the relationship between two people. It depends upon the qualities of both to make a whole, and these qualities can be different in different relationships. So a stone that works in one way for your friend may not work in quite the same way with you, or even in the same way as it did with you under different circumstances. To find which stone is right for you at any one time, you must spend a few moments connecting with the stones. Hold them, one at a time, in your hand and see how you feel. Try out a selection, and work with the one that feels most in tune with the way you need to progress. For example, if you feel tired and depressed then an old favourite, amethyst, may not be right for you this time, as it is a transforming stone and could be too changeable for your mood. Try rose quartz first to calm and clear your emotions or malachite to clear your mind and raise your energy levels. However, amethyst could be the right stone if you need to make decisions that could bring change into your life.

A word of caution – if you have any mental health problems crystals can trigger unwanted reactions.

A selection of crystals

Rose quartz   **Amethyst**   **Citrine**   **Sodalite**   **Turquoise**

 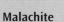

Quartz   **Malachite**   **Garnet**   **Opal**   **Tiger eye**

 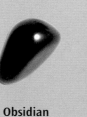

Jade   **Obsidian**   **Jet**   **Amber**   **Carnelian**

Here are a few crystals you might like to try. These descriptions are not comprehensive, merely a guide.

■ *Rose quartz* Calming, cooling influence, releases negativity.
■ *Amethyst* Balances the mental, emotional, and physical bodies, good for life-changing decisions.
■ *Citrine* Balancing, used for aligning the chakras and harmonizing the yin and yang energies.
■ *Sodalite* Aids logical thought, releases confusion, good for group work.
■ *Turquoise* Strengthens and harmonizes the chakras, facilitates communication and intuition.
■ *Quartz* Used for healing, protection, space-clearing. Dispels static electricity. Brings clarity of mind.
■ *Malachite* Clears the mind, aids logical thought processes.
■ *Garnet* Increases steadiness of thought and action, dependability, and orderliness.
■ *Opal* Intensifies powers of perception, awakens creativity. Best used with a protective stone such as carnelian to temper its excesses.

■ *Tiger eye* Opens you to awareness of your true needs and the needs of others. Releases relationship fears, encourages openness toward others.
■ *Jade* Brings gentle peace and harmony to mind and spirit. Enhances intuition. Encourages psychic awareness and receptivity.
■ *Obsidian* Helps to develop inner vision and clarity. Protective. Helps you to find strength in adversity.
■ *Jet* Very protective, calms the mind, dispels unnecessary fears, reduces depression, enhances stability.
■ *Amber* Clears energy, lightens moods, opens you to unconditional love.
■ *Carnelian* Neutralizes negative feelings, encourages loving feelings toward all. Very useful if you wish to move on to working with more dynamic stones as it protects you from the initial rush of enthusiasms and excesses often generated by them.

CHAPTER TWO

Preparation for the day

Plan to get up half an hour or so earlier than you usually do. Waking up slowly, instead of leaping out of bed at the last minute will give your body and mind the opportunity to synchronize. Your muscles will have time to warm up and your mind will clear in readiness for whatever the day brings.

Begin your day before you get out of bed with some stretches and energy-clearing stroking. Then indulge in some energizing massage in your shower. Combine this with a mind- and body-clearing meditation and you will be powered up even before you've had breakfast.

Play games while you are dressing. Feel the action of every muscle, every fibre, every cell. Make it a dance. Be aware of all that you can see, feel the colours. Try to hear every birdsong, the fridge starting up, passing cars. Pretend you are writing a TV script. Describe to yourself everything around you. If you do this often enough you will become bored with the same descriptions and you'll start to find greater depths in everything. This simple exercise will develop your powers of observation and speed up your ability to think in multiple ways.

Appreciate every mouthful of your breakfast. This not only encourages sufficient chewing to start off the digestive process, but you taste more of your food. Try to find all of the different flavours within your meal.

If you need to lose a few pounds, appreciation of the food you are chewing helps to quell the habit of eating more than you really need as it gives your body time to register the amount of food you have swallowed.

Starting the day calmly means that you are less likely to forget the important things that you need to take with you. There will be no last-minute panics. Your day will be organized, productive, and stimulating.

Wake-up routine

Have you ever thrown your feet and calves into a cramp by stretching through to your toes just as you wake up in the morning? By stretching with awareness you can avoid this painful occurrence.

This routine is a very gentle but effective way of waking up your body. Begin before you get out of bed.

NOTES AND SUGGESTIONS

Perform the movements slowly. Breathe in on each stretch and imagine the breath reaching deep within as it follows the stretch. When stretching your legs, be aware of any cramping reaction in your feet or calves and relax your body if you feel this happening.

Always continue breathing in as you tense your muscles and out as you relax.

STRETCHING & STROKING

1. Lie on your back, with your arms above your head. Breathe in and stretch through to your elbows. Breathe out and straighten your arms. On the next breath continue the stretch to your wrists, then ease it out into your fingers. Breathe out into your fingers. Take your awareness back to your shoulders and, in one smooth movement, extend the stretch all the way up to your fingertips, following the ripple of muscles with your mind and your breath .

2. Take your awareness to the back of your neck and ease the stretch out again, following with your breath. This time move it up through your neck and scalp to the top of your head. Relax.

3. Go back to your neck and stretch all your arm and back muscles smoothly upward through your arms and downward to the tops of your legs without tensing your abdominals. Relax.

4. Breathe in and stretch all of the muscles down your front, rippling your abdominal muscles. Relax.

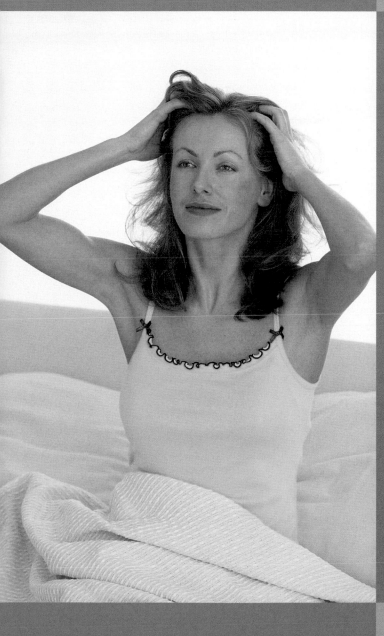

5. Take the stretch down your legs to your heels, stretching your body slowly and fully before taking the movement down to your toes. Keep the tension at your heels as you stretch your feet out. Hop out of bed and place your hands on top of your head. With your fingertips, stroke swiftly and lightly down your face and up the back of your head a few times. With loose fingers, scratch your whole head (see left).

6. Run your fingertips down the front of your body and up the sides as far toward your back as you can reach. Repeat a few times.

7. Run down the front of your legs to the toes and up the back of your legs. Repeat.

8. Stand still, inhaling, holding, and exhaling, each for a count of five. Repeat for ten cycles.

9. Relax, breathing normally.

Tao Yinn and tapping routine

This routine is based in the tradition of the Tao Yinn. It fills your body with energy and clears your mind for the day ahead. You can do the complete routine using only open hands, fingertips, or closed fists, or you can vary it according to the area being worked. Stand with your body held loosely around a central thread that runs up from your feet, through your body, and out the crown of your head. Allow your breath to deepen and feel your heart rate slowing. Feel a connection with the earth. Inhale and pull the breath from far out in the universe into your body. Exhale and push the breath deep down into the earth. Repeat this for a few moments, until you feel you are at one with all. Try to keep your awareness of the connection open throughout the exercise.

1. Start by placing your open hands flat on the top of your head. Close your fists and tap sharply over your head (see left) and down your face, working lightly over your eyes. Repeat three or four times, ending at your chin.

2. Beat down your neck, around the back of your neck, and up to the crown of your head.

3. Open your hands and gently slap them down over your face. Repeat this three or four times, ending with closed fists at the throat.

4. Beat with one fist across to the opposite shoulder (see right) and down the inside of your arm to your hand. Beat back up the outside of that arm and across your upper chest. Change hands and work in the same way across to the other side. Repeat this cycle three or four times.

5. Beat with both fists down your sternum (breastbone) to

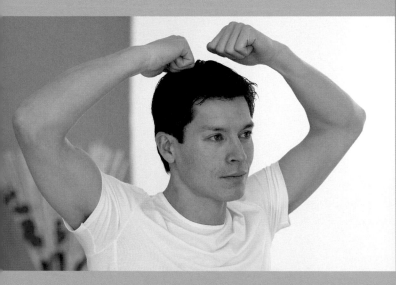

your abdomen. Then beat in a clockwise circle around your abdomen. Repeat this cycle three times.

6. Beat with both fists down your chest and abdomen to the tanden (two finger widths below your navel).

7. Work across to your back and, with the back of your fists, beat up as far as you can reach. Beat with one fist over your upper back and shoulder as far back as you can reach.

8. Change hands and work the other side of your upper back and shoulder. Each time you do this, try to extend your reach farther back.

9. Come back to your throat and repeat the cycle (steps 5 to 8) three or four times, ending at the tanden.

10. Beat with your fists down the front of your legs to your feet, then up the back of your legs to the top of your thighs. Repeat three or four

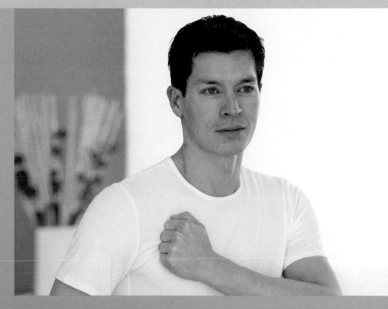

times, ending at your feet.

11. Allow your body to hang in this position for a few moments. Relax your whole body into this, but if you experience any cramp or discomfort come out of the hanging position.

12. Slowly straighten up, with your eyes closed, putting your awareness into the top of your head. Observe any sensations,

feelings, or emotions.

13. Move your awareness down into your chest and observe once again. Do this for three slow breaths.

14. Move your awareness into your abdomen, observe for three breaths. Put your awareness into your strong legs. Take three breaths.

15. Slowly open your eyes. Notice how alive, vibrant, but totally calm you feel.

Breathing

Breathing keeps us alive, yet we don't think about it until we suddenly have to change our rhythm. It oxygenates our minds and bodies. It is necessary for cellular renewal and mental function, and releases the energy stored within our cells. It also detoxifies our bodies – about 80 per cent of the toxins in our system are eliminated through the breath. It can be used to alter our state of consciousness – hyperventilation and reduced oxygen supply to the brain can both affect our perception of reality.

Therapies such as rebirthing, which make use of breathing techniques to increase or decrease the oxygen levels in the brain, can affect ancient memory function, our emotions and feelings, and even our basic attitudes and behaviour patterns.

During the average day we use only our upper lungs, but if we do breathing exercises we use more of our lungs, enlarging their capacity by stretching the fibrous material of which they are made, enabling us to clear out any build-up of dead tissue and toxins, and draw in a greater oxygen supply.

Regular practice of breathing routines will also help with massage. As you move around your partner your breathing will adjust to your energy expenditure and there will be no puffing, jerking, or gasping, just smooth movement and rhythm.

Here is a modified form of an ancient Tantric breathing exercise that builds up and releases a high energy burst within us. It is sometimes known as the "violet breath" or "circular breath".

TANTRIC BREATHING EXERCISE

1. Stand straight, but relaxed, with your knees slightly bent and your eyes closed. Breathe deeply during the whole sequence. Observe your breathing. Feel your lungs working smoothly and efficiently.
2. Place the tip of your tongue just behind your upper front teeth. This closes the gap between the conceptual vessel, which runs from your lower lip, down the front of your body to the Hui Yin point just behind the genitals, and the governing vessel, which runs from the Hui Yin point, up the centre of your back, over the top of your head to your upper lip.
3. Put your awareness into the Hui Yin point. As you inhale, visualize your breath moving up the governing vessel, over the top of your head to meet the conceptual vessel at the tip of your tongue. As you exhale, visualize your breath moving

down the conceptual vessel
to the Hui Yin point.
4. Follow this breath for
three or four cycles, ending
back at the Hui Yin point.
As you end the last cycle on
an out-breath, visualize a
powerful energy moving with
the breath. Pull this energy
up through the governing
vessel and down through
the conceptual vessel.
5. Repeat this flow
for ten breaths, then relax
and open your eyes.

Shower & bath massage

Combining massage with your shower or bath is very beneficial. Many therapies, such as Watsu and hydrotherapy, use the healing power of water, stretching, and massage to relieve various conditions. Stiff muscles and joints, sluggish blood and lymph circulation, poor elimination of toxins, constipation, and many more complaints can be helped through the use of hot and cold water sprays.

IN THE SHOWER

If you wish to use essential oils with a shower it is best to massage the oil into your body first, relax, and have a cup of herbal tea. After about twenty minutes, have a shower. This gives the oils time to soak into your skin and they don't get washed away in the shower.

Hot water is initially stimulating and then relaxing. Cold water is invigorating and toning. Warm water makes you drowsy. Alternating the temperature of your shower revives your whole body.

To massage your body under a shower it is best to use a hand-held unit as this enables you to utilize the full force of the spray close to the showerhead. It will also help if you use a bath or shower seat so that you can more easily raise your feet to spray the soles.

IN THE BATH

Bath massage is relaxing and stimulating, and certain forms of massage, such as underwater massage and massage in conjunction with mineral soaks, can treat a variety of conditions.

To get the best out of a massage in your bath,

SHOWER MASSAGE

1. Run hot water over your whole body. Beginning with your feet, thoroughly massage all over each foot with strong kneading, joint rotations, squeezing, and pinching. Follow your massaging hand with the water spray.
2. Move slowly up to your calves, massaging with strong kneading and squeezing in an upward direction. This helps the natural flow of blood and lymph. Continue all the way up your legs, front, and back in the same manner, following the massage with the water.
3. Work up your abdomen, then work your chest, neck, face, and back.
4. Switch to cold water. Use a scrubbing brush in firm, circular movements, working from your feet to your head, taking care with the more delicate tissues.
5. Return to the hot water and, using your fingertips, scrub over your body with firm rotating movements.
6. Finish with an invigorating cold spray.

combine it with oils or place a small muslin bag filled with porridge oats under the running hot water tap. This is very good for skin complaints such as dry, sensitive skin, eczema, or psoriasis. You can use this with five drops of lavender and five drops of chamomile.

For a relaxing bath after a hard day use three drops of chamomile, three drops of geranium, and two drops of patchouli.

For an invigorating bath use three drops of rosemary and three drops of lemon.

BATH MASSAGE

Massage your body from the feet up, as in the shower sequence. This is incredibly relaxing but if you feel you need to wake up your body and mind, you could follow the bath with a refreshing cold shower.

Sweeping

Sweeping moves any surface energy congestion that has collected over your body, causing sluggishness.

NOTES AND SUGGESTIONS
Your hands may feel as if they are coated in cotton wool. This feeling is caused by a build-up of static energy. Visualize a deep hole opening in the earth and vigorously flick off the coating into the hole.

Repeat all the movements in this sequence three to four times.

1. Put both hands on your face and move them swiftly upward over your face and head, then down to the back of your neck (see left).
2. Place one hand on your opposite shoulder at the base of your neck and sweep it down to your fingertips. Repeat with the other hand.
3. Place both hands on your chest and sweep down the front of your body.
4. Put your hands as far up as you can reach on your back and sweep down.
5. Place both hands on the top of one leg and sweep down to your feet. Repeat with the other leg.
6. Stand relaxed, knees slightly bent, arms by your sides. Shake your head loosely from side to side.
7. Grasp the hair on the top of your head, close to the scalp, and shake it vigorously. Repeat with the hair at the sides and back of your head.
8. Drop your arms. Take several deep breaths, visualizing the air moving down to the soles of your feet on the in-breath and roaring up from your feet and out the top of your head on the out-breath. Do this for five to ten breaths.

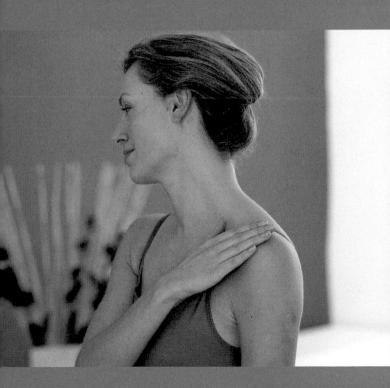

Shaking

Shaking vibrates every cell in our bodies, forcing them to pull in oxygen and nutrients and squeeze out waste matter. It improves circulation and frees up your breathing. It also activates the release of energy within each cell, powering up your mind and body.

NOTES AND SUGGESTIONS
The movement is swift and small. Imagine you are connected to a surging electrical current.

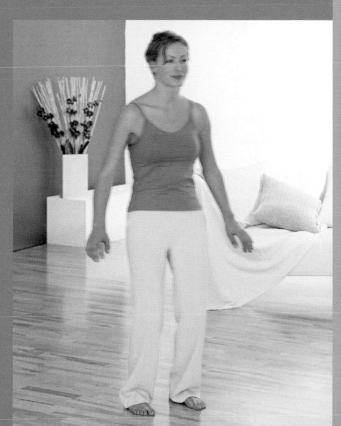

1. Allow your breathing to relax. Put your awareness into the soles of your feet. Shake your feet, gently at first, then more vigorously. Bring the shaking up into your legs. Feel every cell of your feet and legs moving. Bring it up from your legs into your body. Feel all your internal organs shaking.
2. Take the shaking into your hands and arms, feeling the vibration travel from fingertips to shoulders.
3. Move the shaking into your neck and head, feeling the zinging vibrations.
4. Take your awareness back down to your feet and move it slowly up through your body, keeping in touch with the vibration of every cell. Try to identify and move with every cell.
5. As you reach your head, drop your awareness back down to your feet. Keep this cycle going for about five turns, then relax.
6. Allow the shaking to subside. Breathe in long, slow breaths. Don't try to do or be anything, just feel the existence of every cell in your body.
7. When you feel ready, bring yourself back to a state of full awareness.

Ailments and their pressure points

■ *Anxiety, panic attacks* If you are under pressure at work you may find that your levels of anxiety rise or you may even suffer a panic attack. To help in these situations place your fingertips on a pressure point at the centre of your sternum, CV17. Breathe slowly and deeply, and visualize a calming blue cloud around you. After a few moments you will feel your anxiety draining away. To maintain a calm and centred outlook on life it is worthwhile investing 15 to 20 minutes each day in a soothing massage and meditation, and taking regular exercise to boost your oxygen levels. You will find that recurrence of the attacks will decrease. H7, on the wrist, is also a good calming point.

■ *Backache* Emotional stress as well as poor posture can aggravate lower back problems. For quick relief, ask a partner or colleague to help. (Do not use this massage if the problem is a medical condition.) Sit on a stool with your elbows on your knees or straddle an armless chair, facing its back. Have your partner place their hands on your lower back, with the heels about two finger widths from your spine and their fingers

angled at about 45 degrees. Ask them to lean in with all of their weight and 'walk' up and down your back, hand over hand, for a few moments. This will loosen any tension. There are also pressure points that you can use – B23, which are located just up from waist level and about two finger widths out from either side of the spine, and B47, which are about two finger widths to the outer sides of B23. They could be quite tender, so use them with care. Use fists, fingers, or thumbs to apply a firm pressure for a few moments.

■ *Breathing difficulties* There are several pressure points that will help relieve breathing problems. On your hand there are two, L9 and L10. These are near your thumbs. L9 is at the base of the inside of your thumb and L10 is about two finger widths up along the thumb bone. Briskly rub these points on both hands, for a few moments. Some breathing difficulties are caused by toxin build-up within your body. To help to move these, massage points B13, K27, and L1 regularly. B13 are situated two finger widths either side of the spine and one finger width below the level of the shoulder blades. K27 are in the hollow just below the collar-bone and either side of your sternum. L1 are just inward from each shoulder joint and three finger widths below the sternum. As breathing problems can be triggered by emotional stress the treatment for anxiety can be beneficial.

■ *Colds* There are many pressure points around the face and head that will help drain a cold and clear the sinuses. GB20 are at the base of the skull and about two finger widths either side of the spine, in the dimply area. Strong massage here will quickly help to clear a cold. GV16, which is in the centre between the two GB20's, is a very good point for other symptoms such as headache and stiff necks. For the sinuses, apply pressure to B2, in the inner corner of the eyebrows. Pressure to the LI20 points either side of your nose, will also help your sinuses.

■ *Hangovers* You will need to encourage the body to move the toxins of alcohol and help the blood flow to the brain. Massage strongly into LI4, which is in the fleshy area between the thumb and first finger of each hand. The points for eye strain will help with headache; these are B2, ST3, and GV24.5, the latter of which is in the centre of the fore-head. A gentle head massage may help but you may feel too delicate for this.

■ *Insomnia* A long leisurely bath with lavender oil, a cup of peppermint tea, a full body massage, or a head massage, concentrating on your upper back and neck, will help to release any physical and emotional problems that stop you getting a good night's sleep.You can also massage some of the anaesthetic points given in the general pain section (see p.42), especially LI4. Massaging the ear-lobes can also help to relax the mind.

■ *Stomach problems* As a preventive measure, regular massage on CV12, half-way between the navel and the base of the sternum is very useful, but avoid this point if you have just eaten or if you have high blood pressure or heart disease. About two finger widths below the navel is CV6 – massage this point if you are suffering from digestive upset, abdominal pain, or constipation.

Refer to pp.16–19 and 42–3 in order to locate the various pressure points.

■ *General pain* As well as massaging
the painful area with thumb and
palm rubbing, there are pressure
points for the root cause of the pain.
For the upper body, massage with
strong rotations or continuous
pressure on: point LI4, which is
found in the fleshy area between the
thumb and first finger of each hand;
GV24.5, at the bridge of the nose
between the eyes; GB20, at the base
of the skull, two finger widths either
side of the spine; and GV16, at the
top of the spine where it meets the
head. For lower body pain you can
massage ST36, which is found about
four finger widths below the
kneecap and one finger width from
the bone toward the outer area of
the leg. If you press on this spot and
move your foot you should feel a
movement in the muscle. It can also
feel quite painful under pressure.
K3, on the inside of the ankle in the
dimply area between the bone and
the Achilles tendon, is another good
pressure point, as is B60, which can
be found on the outside of the
ankle at the same level.

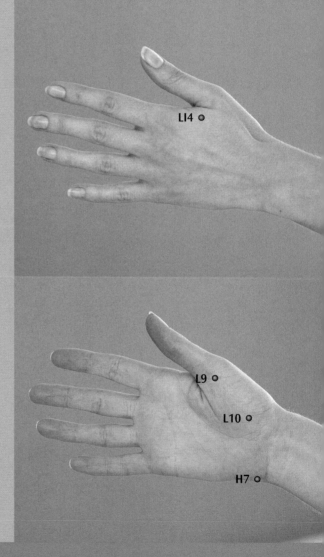

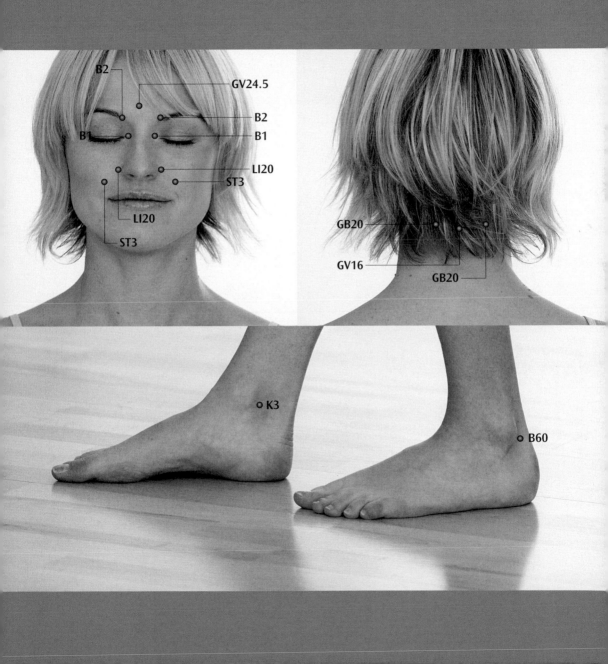

Chakra meditation

I shall be using the term "chakra" as it is commonly understood, to mean an energy centre of the body and aura. There are many more chakras within the human energy system than the seven main ones that are usually worked. Tiny chakras are found throughout the body and aura. We are literally surrounded by hundreds of these minor energy centres, each of which is connected with every other chakra. In disciplines such as Shiatsu, which recognizes meridians with various tsubos (pressure points) along their lengths, many of these minor chakras are worked. Those who use energy healing systems also connect with the chakras within the auras to detect and treat the various disturbances that can cause ill health.

This chakra meditation is very energizing so it is a good idea to do it in the morning or at midday rather than in the evening. If you practise the sequence regularly you will find that it has a cumulative effect which will help to build your stamina, calm your mind, open your awareness, and develop your intuition. It will strengthen your healing powers and allow you to give more to your partner during massage without draining your own energy supplies. Allow yourself to be with the power of the light. It may feel strange at first – light-headedness and slight dizziness are normal reactions. If you wish you can do the meditation sitting down until you become used to the physical sensations that accompany it.

Your room should be comfortably warm and well aired, perhaps with a scented oil burning and low, soft music playing, or silence, if you prefer.

1. Stand with your feet about shoulder-width apart, your knees flexible and slightly bent, and your arms hanging loosely by your sides. Breathe slowly and deeply, but without directing your breath at this stage.
2. Put your attention into the earth beneath your feet. Feel it as a living entity. Connect with the life of all things.
3. Move your awareness deep into the earth, to the fire energy of its centre. Feel that connection moving up through your body and out from the top of your head.
4. Slowly move your attention up through the air above you. Feel the connection between the earth and the universe.
5. Move your awareness to the farthest parts of the universe. You are now within a channel that leads from the centre of the earth out to the universe. Visualize the sun and the moon in a straight line with you in the channel between them.

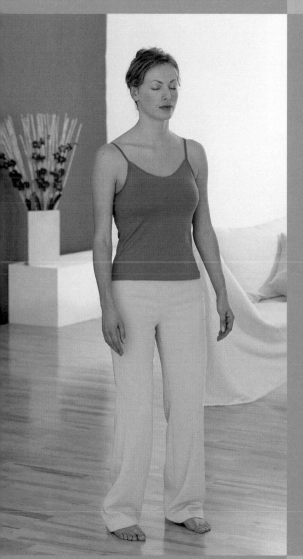

*6. Breathe in – see a light
coming from the universe
to the sun.
Breathe out – feel the sun
absorbing the light and
growing brighter.
Breathe in – see the bright
light moving from the sun
to the moon.
Breathe out – feel the moon
absorbing the light and
growing brighter.
Breathe in – see the light
moving from the moon to a
point, a chakra, about one
metre (3 feet) above your
head. This is your
transpersonal point.
Breathe out – feel this
chakra glowing with a bright
white light. You may now
feel the power of the energy
moving within your aura.
Breathe in – see the light
enter the top of your head,
your crown chakra.
Breathe out – feel your
crown chakra absorbing the
power and glowing with a
violet light.
Breathe in – see the light
move down into your third
eye (brow) chakra.*

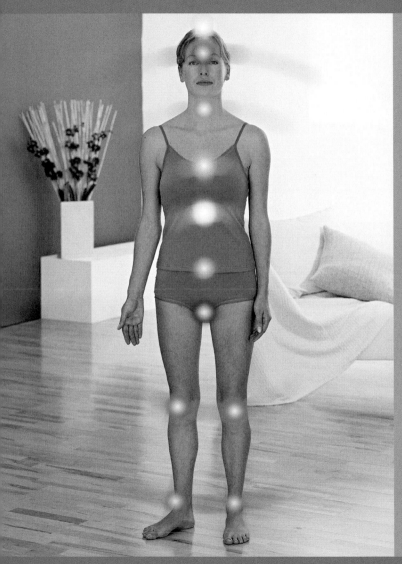

Breathe out – feel your third eye chakra glowing with an indigo light.
Breathe in – see the light continue to move down to your throat chakra.
Breathe out – feel your throat chakra glowing with a soft blue light.
Breathe in – see the light branch out and move across your shoulders and down your arms, into your hands and palm chakras.
Breathe out – feel your arms and hands filling with a silver light. Open your hands. Feel your fingers extending down into the earth to open the channel and complete this connection.
Breathe in – see the light move down your body to your heart chakra.
Breathe out – feel your heart chakra glowing with a green light. (You may also have a sense of pink or turquoise with this chakra – some people have become aware of another chakra opening just above the heart chakra.

If you feel this, just allow the light to fill the whole area of your upper chest.)
Breathe in – see the light move down to the solar plexus chakra.
Breathe out – feel your solar plexus glowing with a yellow light.
Breathe in – see the light move down to your sacral chakra (hara).
Breathe out – feel your sacral chakra glowing with an orange light.
Breathe in – see the light continue to move down to your base chakra.
Breathe out – feel your base chakra glowing with a vibrant red light.
Breathe in – see the light move down to your knees (minor chakra).
Breathe out – feel your knees glowing with a dark holly-green light.
Breathe in – see the light move down to your feet (minor chakra).
Breathe out – feel your feet glowing with a dark russet-brown light.

Breathe in – see the light move down to your earth point (this is a minor chakra) about one metre (3 feet) below your feet.
Breathe out – feel this point glowing with a black light (the opposite and balance to your transpersonal point).
Breathe in – see the light move down to the centre of the earth. Move your attention back out to the universe once more.
Breathe out – feel the light streaming down from the universe, through your chakras, gathering all of the colours as it goes. The light moves down to the centre of the earth.
Breathe in – see a fountain of light spray out all around you from the centre of the earth, lighting up all of the hundreds of chakras within your aura as it moves in a vast ball of light that encompasses the universe and all within it.
7. Continue breathing and moving this energy ball from the universe, down through

your body to the centre of the earth and back to the universe, lighting up and strengthening your whole being, for about seven slow, smooth breaths.
8. Slowly, on the final out-breath, ending far out in the universe, start to close down the column of light. As you breathe in, feel the light dimming. Close down all of the chakras within your aura.
Breathe evenly with long, slow breaths.
9. Draw the light up the column through each chakra (don't tighten up at this stage, the chakras need some movement), closing them gently like a flower at evening until you reach your transpersonal point, a metre (3 feet) above your head. Then gather all of the energy and move it back down into your sacral chakra.
10. Finally, gently close your sacral chakra.
Allow your breathing to return to normal and come back to full awareness.

CHAPTER THREE

Massage on the move

The journey to and from your place of work can be a trying time. Crowded roads, buses, and trains create and hold high levels of aggressive energy. However, you could also see your journey as a little break between home and work where you can enjoy the changing scenery, listen to music, talk to people.

If you are driving use every stop, tailback, and snarl-up as an opportunity to refresh your levels of calm, and stretch your hands to ease out that tense grip. Shrug your shoulders and roll your head to ease tired neck muscles. A small cushion placed at your lower back will help to support you and make your sitting position more comfortable.

If you travel on crowded trains and buses, your legs and back may ache through inactivity, and if you are strap-hanging, your arms may also need some help to release any cramps. Moving your weight slightly every few moments will help your circulation and will slide muscle tissues over each other, releasing any build-up of toxins within the fibres.

If you travel in a closed vehicle, you keep breathing the same tired air, which will contain a higher than normal level of carbon dioxide and bacteria. The best way to combat these problems is to walk as far as you can during any journey. Park your car at a car park farther away than usual from your place of work, get on and off trains and buses at stops a little farther from work, enjoy the breeze in your hair, and feel a part of your surroundings. If you have to travel by plane, take regular walks up and down the aisles to clear your mind and body of the staleness, stress, and tension of travelling.

The importance of breathing

Every thought we have influences every breath we take. In a tense or even exciting situation our brains and our bodies need more oxygen. This releases the energy that enables us to think faster and respond rapidly. As this function is more under the control of our autonomic nervous system than our conscious direction, it can easily move into overdrive.

Stress, fear, fun, or just physical exertion all trigger a similar response. We breathe more rapidly, our heart rate increases, and our bodies prepare for action. All of this pulls extra oxygen into our bloodstream, making it more alkaline. If this extra oxygen isn't used up it can cause physical problems such as dizziness, fainting, tingling and numbness in your scalp and hands, and even visual disturbances. This is the body's way of shutting down to reduce the rate at which oxygen is consumed. Your conscious mind interprets these symptoms as anxiety and panic, which is why even mildly stressful situations, such as those that arise every day when we are travelling, can induce what we consider to be irrational fears. At this point we need less oxygen and more carbon dioxide. Well-controlled breathing will maintain a good balance of carbon dioxide and oxygen in the bloodstream.

Doing a few breathing exercises before or during massage will help to oxygenate the muscles, thus releasing muscle tension during a relaxing massage. Good breath control also helps to release toxins and waste products within the muscle structure, which can then be carried away by the blood.

Alternate nostril breathing

This technique calms the mind, reduces facial pain, clears the sinuses, and relaxes the jaw. It helps you to focus mentally and physically, facilitating concentration, and calms over-stimulating thoughts.

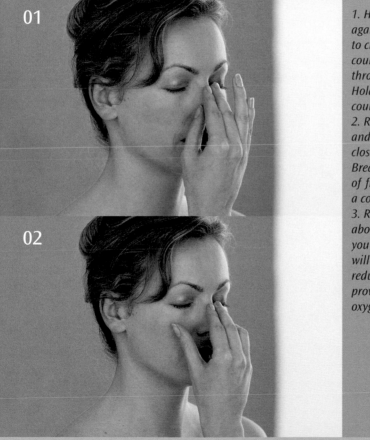

01

02

1. Hold your right thumb against your right nostril to close it and, slowly, to a count of five, breathe in through your left nostril (01). Hold your breath for a count of five.
2. Release your right nostril and hold your left nostril closed with your finger (02). Breathe out for a slow count of five. Hold your breath for a count of five.
3. Repeat steps 1 and 2 about ten times, or more if you feel you need to. This will help to clear your head, reduce your anxieties, and provide a good supply of oxygen to your bloodstream.

Walking to work

Many people who work long hours can feel that they are missing out on life. Days come and go in a blur of meetings, decisions, dashing from one crisis to the next, and battling with confusion. While life is dancing all around them, they can feel very disconnected.

Walking to work, even in bad weather, can help to reconnect you, and it's a most enjoyable way to travel. You can breathe fresh air, get some refreshing exercise, and travel slowly enough to appreciate the changing seasons and all that is going on around you. If you live at some distance from your place of work, get off the bus a few stops before your destination and walk the rest of the way.

Walking with awareness can be used to give yourself an internal massage. By putting your awareness into your body and feeling exactly how your bones, muscles, tendons, and internal organs are moving, you can actively direct minute movements that stimulate a massaging of fibre on fibre. If you walk with awareness you can help your body to build up fitness, eliminate waste products, oxygenate tissues, increase flexibility, and relax your entire being.

Give yourself the time to really enjoy your walk. Allow time to make detours to new and interesting places, such as river banks, different market places, across fields, and through woodland. If you have to walk through streets, try different ways of reaching your destination – walk through a city park or along a canal bank. This can help you to see life fresh and new each day. Talk to people – even in the busy rush of morning there are interesting ideas to be explored, and seeing friends and making new ones helps to keep the channels of communication open.

While you walk, observe the ways you move your limbs, balance, and shift your weight as you take each step. Feel your back muscles – are they stooped? Change your posture, carry your weight high, imagine your whole weight as a ball above your head, and look around you instead of at the ground. This will help to rebalance and realign your whole body and pull energizing fresh air deep into your lungs.

Breathe deeply – even in a busy street, with passing traffic, deep breathing will help to clear your mind and remove toxins from your body. Over 80 per cent of detoxing happens through the breath. Good levels of oxygen are also necessary for the efficient release of energy within the body and for effective brain work.

You can also try a walking meditation. This is simply stilling your mind and being totally aware of moving one step at a time as you travel through space. Synchronize your breathing with your steps. Bring a smooth rhythm to all of your movements. Put your awareness into each tiny movement, but at the same time keep contact with everything that is going on around you. Even walking has its dangers.

Arriving at work after walking is very different from arriving after driving or travelling on a crowded train or bus. You feel more alive and ready for the day's challenges, rather than tired and headachy.

Massage for travelling

HEAD MASSAGE
Headaches are common travelling complaints.
Low oxygenation, stale cabin air, immobility, and
altitude can all adversely affect you. To help to
restore the balance of pressure within your head,
clear your sinuses, and help to ease tired eyes,
try this pressure massage.

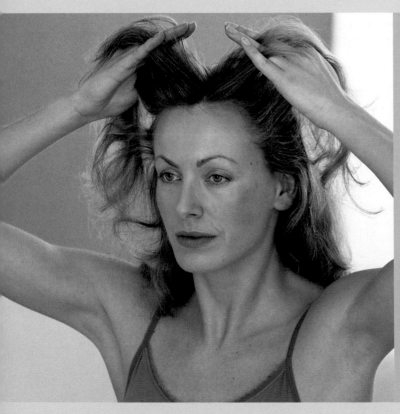

1. Place your thumbs just under your jaw, by your ears, and drop the weight of your head on to them. Hold for a count of five and release.
2. Move your thumbs a finger width down your jaw in the direction of your chin and drop your head on to them again and hold. Repeat all along your jaw line.
3. Place the fingers of each hand under your cheekbones, so that your little fingers are either side of your nose.
4. Drop the weight of your head on to your fingers. Hold for a slow count of ten and release. Breathe slowly through your nose. Repeat this three times.

NECK MASSAGE

To ease an aching neck, hold your head with both hands and toss your head loosely from side to side. Try to take your head to its limit of movement. This should be a gentle action. Keep full control of the weight of your head with your hands at all times. Try to relax your neck and shoulders more each time your head moves.

1. Place the fingers of both hands on the back of your neck, either side of your spine and running down the length of your neck vertebra.
2. With strong rotations work your fingers firmly into the muscles of the neck, for a count of five.
3. Move your fingers sideways by one finger width and again work firmly into your neck. Repeat twice more and then relax your neck.
4. Drop your head forward, swinging it slowly from side to side to loosen the muscles.
5. Hook your thumbs into the hollows located at both sides of the spine at the top of your neck.
6. Firmly push in an upward direction while slowly moving your head back on to your thumbs. Hold this position for a count of ten. Release and relax.
7. Rub the whole of the back of your neck firmly with your knuckles.

5. Close your eyes. Place your thumbs under your eyebrows either side of your nose. Drop the weight of your head on to your thumbs. Hold for a slow count of ten. Release, screw up your eyes, and hold for a count of ten. Repeat this three times.
6. Place all the fingers of both hands in a line along your hairline so that your little fingers are touching. Press firmly into your scalp and hold for a count of ten. Move your fingers about a finger width back toward the crown of your head and repeat the pressure.
7. Repeat the pressure in one finger width intervals until you have reached the crown of your head.

8. Place your fingers in a vertical line at the sides of your head, in line with your ears, and repeat the pressure massage backward until your fingers meet at the back of your head.
9. Run your fingers through the hair over the top of your head. Close your fingers up together so that you are holding a good handful of hair in each hand and pull firmly out from the scalp so that your hair is slowly running under tension through your fingers (see left). Repeat this pull in a perpendicular direction, all over your head.

SHOULDER MASSAGE

For shoulder aches, place your left hand on your right shoulder, just under your right ear, and grasp firmly (see below). Hold the pinch for a count of three. Move down your shoulder about a palm width and repeat. Repeat this along your other shoulder. There are some very powerful pressure points along your shoulders which may be painful, but it is very good to work them firmly. Do not use this technique over the middle of your shoulders, GB21, if you are pregnant.

1. Raise your right arm above your head and take hold of the elbow with your left hand.
2. Drop your right hand down behind your head. Exert pressure with your left hand to extend the stretch and hold for about 20 seconds. Repeat on the other side.
3. Shrug your shoulders several times up and down and then backward and forward several times.
4. Raise both hands in the air. Cross them over and try to grasp as far down one arm as you can. While holding with one hand, try to creep the fingers of the other hand farther down the arm, then hold firmly. Then do the same with the other hand. Hold the final position for a count of five.
5. Relax.

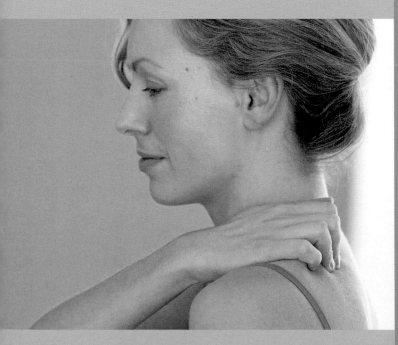

ARM AND HAND MASSAGE

When you have finished the shoulder massage, move on down to your arms. Explore the movement of your wrists and hands in all directions.

Hold your wrists in the extreme positions for a count of ten for each movement, and release. Do the same with each of your fingers. This will loosen your wrists and hands and improve their flexibility.

1. Grasp the top of your right arm with your left hand and firmly knead with your fingers and thumb down your arm and into your hand (01). Continue the kneading all over your hand (02).
2. When you reach the end of each finger, firmly pinch the fingertip and pull strongly, then shake vigorously. Repeat with the other arm and hand.

01

02

ABDOMINAL MASSAGE

Travelling often causes stomach upsets. Strange food, tension, and the smell of diesel or aviation fuel can all trigger symptoms of nausea, constipation, and diarrhoea. To combat the smell of fuel a few drops of lavender and frankincense on a tissue or your clothing can help to disguise any unpleasantness and calm you.

Stomach upsets:

Massage with rotations on points ST43 and ST44, which are on the top of your feet, just between your second and third toes (see pp.18–19). They are very close together so if you massage from between your toes to about one finger width below the base of your toes you will be working the correct area. Another two points are ST41, at the centre front of your ankle, and ST36, four finger widths below your kneecap, on the outer side of your leg.

Other digestive disorders:

1. Using your fist, massage in gentle rotations from right to left across the whole of your abdominal area.
2. You can also use 'the wave'. Press with the heel of your right hand on the right side of your stomach and firmly slide across to the left side of your stomach.
3. Roll the pressure along your hand to your fingertips and, gently pressing in with your fingertips, pull your hand back across your stomach. Repeat this all over your stomach area.

BACK MASSAGE

1. Make your hands into fists and hold the knuckles of each hand against your spine as low down your back as you can reach without discomfort.
2. Lean back slightly on to your hands so that you can feel a strong pressure against your spine. Massage into your back for a few moments.
3. Keeping your hands at the same level, move your fists out toward your sides about a palm width and lean back again. Follow this with massage. Repeat across the full width of your back.
4. Go back to your spine to a position about a palm width higher and repeat the leaning back and the massage. Try to raise the level of your fist twice more and repeat the massage. This will loosen an aching back and will also benefit your shoulder flexibility.

LEG AND FOOT MASSAGE
To help avoid deep vein thrombosis (DVT) on long journeys you should start to massage your legs every 20 to 30 minutes from the beginning of your trip.

1. Take your shoes off and use the heel of one foot to massage your other leg strongly, from the top of your foot up to your knee (01). Massage in an upward direction. You can also use your toes and upper foot to massage the back of your calves (02).

2. Then continue by using your hands to massage one leg at a time with a strong kneading action, working in an upward direction, to encourage blood flow back to the body.

3. Continue the kneading massage up over your thighs, working into all of the muscles in that area (03).

CAUTION
Do not work strongly if you suffer from varicose veins.

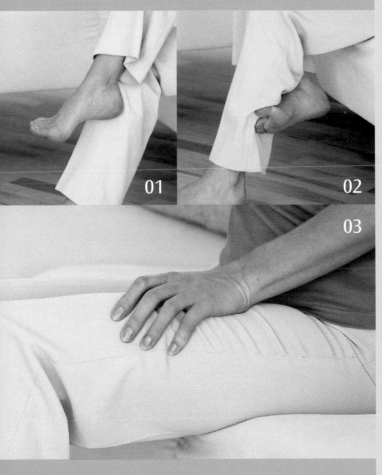

01

02

03

CHAPTER FOUR

Massage at work

It can be difficult to take more than a few moments out of your working day to use massage. The deep benefits of massage have much to do with allowing yourself to forget everything and let go. Even a few moments can be useful when you have a headache, tired eyes, or stiff muscles.

Having finally made it in to work through the rush hour you may already feel wound up, tense, stressed, and unable to face the day until you've had at least three cups of coffee. Resist this impulse.

Find a quiet corner. Bunch your hands into fists and vigorously rub your knuckles from the back of your head to the front, covering your whole head in sweep after energetic sweep. If you still feel tense, continue the knuckling down your neck, across your shoulders, down each arm in turn, down your front, and over your back.

There are some pressure points running down the length of your sternum (breastbone) that can help to clear your breathing if your chest feels tight. Press as hard as you can at the top of your sternum with your index and middle fingers. Hold for a count of ten. Move down about two finger widths and repeat until the end of the sternum.

Work one leg at a time with strong knuckling, using both fists massaging either side of your leg, down to your feet. Repeat over the other leg.

Now use your breath to re-energize your system quickly. Take deep, long, slow breaths. As you breathe in, feel the breath pulling strong invigorating energy up from the centre of the earth. As you breathe out, push this energy into every cell of your being. Continue this breathing cycle for 15 to 20 breaths. If you feel dizzy or light-headed, stop the deep breaths and breathe normally, but continue the visualization until you have completed at least 15 cycles.

Meditation

After a rush hour journey to work you may well feel the need to rid yourself of the hassle of the trip before even trying to think of anything else you have to do.

This meditation connects you to the power of colour. You can begin on any colour of the spectrum. I find that yellow makes a good start. If you are feeling harassed you can move in the red direction, ending in the calming blues and greens. If you need an energy boost, move through the blues toward the reds. Here we shall move in the red direction. You can do this meditation standing or seated.

NOTES AND SUGGESTIONS

Always visualize your colour moving toward you through a mist. As you breathe in, you will feel the colour on which you are meditating deepening. As this happens, feel every changing shade of the colour.

While you are doing the meditation imagine the healing energies working and you will bring the body's self-healing abilities into action. If you are giving a massage you will release the power of the universal healing energies; if you are receiving one you will activate your own healing process, thus increasing the effectiveness of the massage.

1. Close your eyes and imagine that you are surrounded by a golden-yellow egg-shaped mist.
2. Breathe in and feel the colour deepen at the outer edges of the mist.
3. Breathe out and feel the deeper colour moving toward you, filling you with a rich yellow glow.
4. Breathe in and feel the outer edges slowly turning to a clear orange. Be fully aware of this colour, taste it, smell it, feel its touch.
5. Breathe out and feel the colour moving toward you, filling you with an energizing rich orange glow.
6. Breathe in and feel the edges darken to red.
7. Breathe out and feel the deeper colour moving toward you, filling you with an energizing rich red glow.
8. Breathe in and feel the colour changing to a rich purple. Feel the healing purple colour moving toward you.
9. Breathe out and feel the colour moving through you,

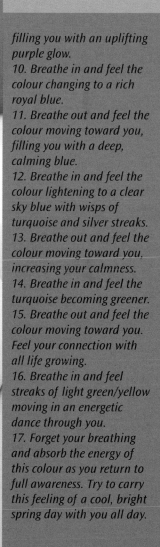

filling you with an uplifting purple glow.

10. Breathe in and feel the colour changing to a rich royal blue.

11. Breathe out and feel the colour moving toward you, filling you with a deep, calming blue.

12. Breathe in and feel the colour lightening to a clear sky blue with wisps of turquoise and silver streaks.

13. Breathe out and feel the colour moving toward you, increasing your calmness.

14. Breathe in and feel the turquoise becoming greener.

15. Breathe out and feel the colour moving toward you. Feel your connection with all life growing.

16. Breathe in and feel streaks of light green/yellow moving in an energetic dance through you.

17. Forget your breathing and absorb the energy of this colour as you return to full awareness. Try to carry this feeling of a cool, bright spring day with you all day.

Coffee break massage

During your coffee break you can refresh your aching shoulders, arms, and hands. This will also help to ward off any tension headaches as it will loosen your upper back muscles. As your hands and arms contain many meridians, you can give your body a tone-up with a little hand and arm massage. Stretching your hands during your coffee break can help to ease any aches and improve their flexibility.

There are several channels running along both the outer and inner areas of your arms, from your fingertips to your upper body. These can be massaged to tone and stimulate not just the muscles and tendons of your arms but also your organs. While massaging your arm, breathe deeply and visualize a warmth moving down into the top of your head, through your body to your hara (lower abdomen), then back up into your arms. Try to see this cycle as a continuous, calming flow of energy.

NOTES AND SUGGESTIONS
TH4 is on the triple heater channel (see pp.16–17) and is very good for wrist pain. The triple heater is not really a specific organ, but a collection of organs that includes your lungs, and your digestive and elimination systems. Working this channel, which runs along your arm from the back of your ring finger up the length of the outside of your arm, can help with any abdominal and lower back pain.

Your middle finger carries the heart protector or pericardium channel, and massaging this point will help to ease any emotional stress, tightness in your chest, and indigestion.

The index finger holds the large intestine channel on its outside and massaging this will help with any abdominal problems such as flatulence, constipation, and diarrhoea.

Your thumb contains the lung channel, which runs up the inside of your hand and arm. L9, on the inside of your wrist, just below your thumb, and L10, located about two finger widths above L9 on your thumb, are very good points to massage if you are experiencing breathing problems (see pp.18–19 and p.42).

H7 is a point on the heart channel (see p.42). Working along both the heart channel and the small intestine channel will help to calm you, boost your energy, and clear your head.

The final stretch (see step 11, p.67) is very good if you have ever broken your hand or wrist as it will help you to regain complete flexibility.

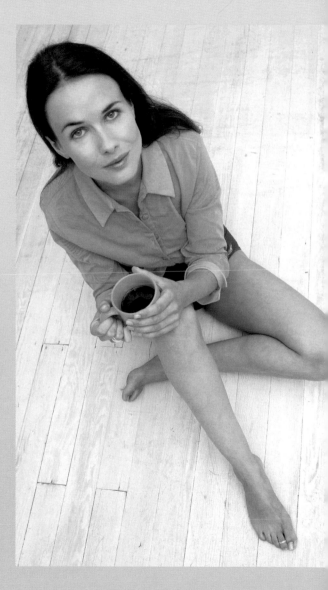

01

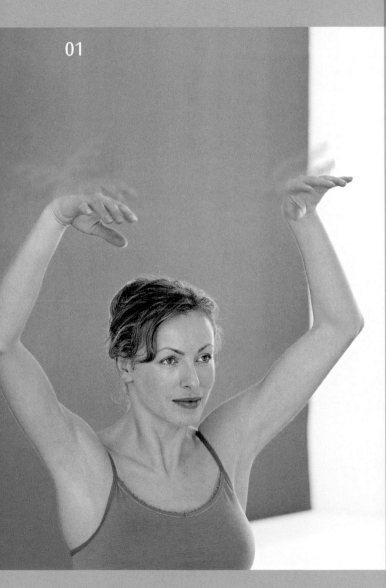

1. Hold your hands above your head for 20–30 seconds. Vigorously shake your fingers while they are still in the air (01). Shake your hands, then your arms, then your shoulders, moving them up and down, back and forth. This will boost the circulation in your hands and arms.

2. Lower the hands and grip one little finger with the thumb and fingers of your other hand, thumb on the top and fingers underneath. With strong pinching and kneading movements, work your way slowly along the outer edge of your hand.

At your wrist, spend a few moments massaging strongly into H7, just where the bones of your little finger meet the bones of your forearm (02). Move along your forearm up to your shoulder (03).

3. Take hold of your ring finger and pinch and knead back along its length. Continue until you reach the joining of the finger bones with the forearm bones and here work with strong thumb rotations into TH4 (see pp. 16–17).
4. Repeat on your other arm.
5. Put your hands together and raise your elbows so that your forearms are at right angles to your hands.
6. Rotate your hands as far as they can go, away from your body. Hold that position for a count of ten.
7. Rotate your hands toward your body, as far as they can go, and again hold for a count of ten.
8. Come back to the centre and, while keeping the heels of your hands together, turn your fingertips toward you and push the heels of your hands away from you. Hold for a count of ten.

9. Come back to the centre. Push your left hand over to the left with your right hand. Make sure your hands make contact all the way down. Hold for a count of ten.
10. Come back to the centre and use your left hand to push your right hand over toward the right. Hold for a count of ten.
11. Lean your elbows on the desk and hold one hand with its palm toward you. Take hold of your little finger with your other hand and drop it back so that you are stretching your little finger back as far as it will go. Don't force the stretch, just allow the weight of your hand to move your finger backward. Hold for a count of ten. Repeat with the rest of your fingers and thumbs.

02

03

Stretching, neck loosening

This is a full body workout which releases waste matter from the system, lubricates the joints, strengthens the muscles, and stretches the tendons. Since every cell in the body renews itself every few weeks, we can accumulate a great deal of waste matter through cellular degeneration and renewal. Inactivity, stress, tension, emotional problems, depression, illness, injury, and self-indulgence also deposit their own rubbish.

In an ideal world we would have perfect bodies, able to renew and refresh every cell without any problems. However, we don't get enough exercise, and we don't eat and drink only that which is good for our minds and bodies. Our thoughts are not based on that which brings good health and well-being to ourselves and our society. We enjoy danger, stress, and excitement. We have problems with relationships which wind us up and drop us from great emotional heights. In general, we treat ourselves very badly. This particularly affects the large muscles of our shoulders and neck. Mental stress immediately creates tension here, which can build up day after day to cause problems with pain and immobility – frozen shoulder, stiff neck, and tired, aching head and arms

Ideally, we should take on board only that which we need and will be of benefit to us. We need to produce energy to allow our minds to work, our bodies to move, and our spirits to create and enjoy. The process of energy production is based in combustion. Oxygen and calories in our food and drink burn to produce energy. This also produces waste matter. The exchange of food for waste products within our blood and lymph fluids should be able to rid our bodies of this waste. However, we tend to habitually abuse our bodies and overload our systems, and – over years – the waste products produced by these abuses and excesses, which our circulatory systems can't disburse, build up within our tissues, causing deposits that can affect our health. These deposits start as a coagulation, move on into a heavier gelatinous substance, and finally harden into a crystalline crust, which can eventually calcify and seriously injure our joints and under-used muscles.

This is where stretching and deep breathing exercises can help. When we stretch, the fibres within our muscles slide over each other. As these fibres slide, constant movement produces a pumping action, which breaks up any deposits within our muscles so that blood and lymph fluid can dissolve and carry away the refuse. Stretching to the fullest extent of our reach works deeply into these fibres, digging out old deposits. Aided by massage, you can go even farther. By breaking down hard-to-dissolve substances and squeezing and massaging them out of the fibres you can shift years of waste build-up, so helping to renew and regenerate your whole being. You feel calmer as your body relaxes into a healthy rhythm, without the strain and stress of having to work overtime trying to maintain a seized-up and clogged system.

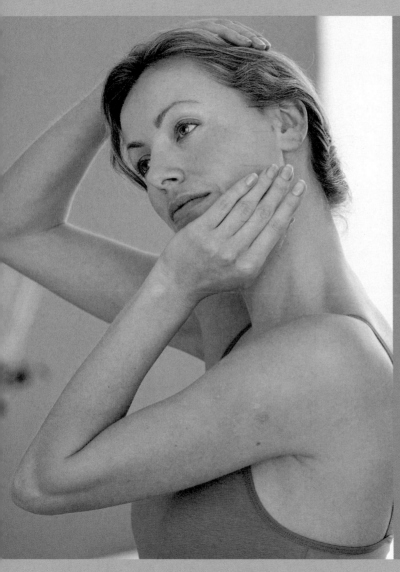

1. Stand with your feet about shoulder-width apart. Raise your arms and reach upward as far as you can. Breathe in deeply and out fully, and increase the stretch. Relax one arm but do not let it drop. Breathe in deeply and out fully and increase the stretch in the other arm.
2. Relax this arm and stretch your other arm. Breathe in deeply and out fully and increase the stretch.
3. Reach up with both arms. Breathe in and, as you let your breath go out, drop forward from your waist and allow your upper body to hang down loosely from your waist for a few slow breaths.
4. Feel the tension gradually draining out of your upper body. Start to swing gently from right to left. Don't force anything, just flop and swing for a count of 20–30. If you feel at all uncomfortable come out of the stretch, but each time you do the exercise, aim to extend your hanging count up to 60.

5. Stand up and stretch your arms out to the sides. Move one arm straight up above your head and allow it to bend at the elbow to drop the hand down behind your head. Swing the other hand up behind your back to meet it. If you can, clasp your fingers. Grip with your fingers as tightly as you can for a count of ten.

6. Release the tension, and then grip again. Repeat three or four times. Change your arms over, so that they are in the opposite position and repeat the stretch.

7. Sit down, allowing your arms to hang by your sides. Raise your shoulders until they meet your ears. Hold for a count of five, then drop them. Repeat this a few times until you can feel that your neck is holding some tension. On the last raise allow your head to drop to one side and, as you lower your shoulders, allow your head to be lowered on to one shoulder.

8. Raise both shoulders. At the top of the movement centre your head, then drop it on to the other shoulder.

9. Lower your shoulders and carry your head down with them. Repeat five times on each side.

10. Drop your head on to your chest. Clasp your hands behind your neck and pull your head farther down. Resist the pull of your arms by tensing your neck. Hold the pull for a count of ten.

11. Release and repeat the neck pull about 5 times or as many times as you can manage without feeling any discomfort or strain. While you have your hands behind your head and your head down, ask a colleague to pull up on your elbows for a few moments.

12. Come out of the stretch. Place your right hand on your neck, just under your left ear. With strong rotation, massage in a line across your shoulder. There are some quite painful spots here which respond well to strong massage. Work back and forth along this line for a few moments, then change hands and repeat along the opposite shoulder.

13. Hold the top left side of your head with your right hand (see left) and place the heel of your left hand on the right side of your chin. Pull gently with your right hand and push with your left, twisting your head round to the left. Hold for a count of 30. Release, bringing your head back to centre. Repeat on the other side.

Dealing with indigestion

Working lunches, stress, and eating on the go can cause your stomach to rebel. For abdominal pains you will need to calm your mind and internal organs to allow them to release their tension.

1. Stand with your hands placed on your abdomen, just below your navel (tanden; see right). Take some deep slow breaths. On the in-breath, visualize a cool light, pale spring green or sky blue, moving into your body with your breath. On the out-breath, visualize this cooling, healing light filling your abdomen.
2. On the next in-breath, draw more of the cooling light into your abdomen, absorbing the pain and discomfort. On the next out-breath, push this light down your legs and out through the soles of your feet.

Continue breathing in this way as you slowly start to massage your stomach.
3. Place the heel of your right hand just under your ribcage on the right hand side. Press in firmly with the heel of your hand and slowly slide it across to the left side of your abdomen. Repeat this four or five times.
4. Move your right hand down about a hand width and repeat the massage.
5. Move your hand down once more and repeat again.
6. Place your left hand on your solar plexus. Hold the thumb and first three fingers of your right hand in a claw,

similar to the tiger's claw (see pp.98–9) but slightly tighter, with approximately 1 cm (1/2 in) distance between each finger.
7. Now starting on the right hand side of your abdomen, massage with small, firm, clockwise rotations, for about four or five rotations on each position. Work slowly, with the intention of dissolving the pain. Cover the whole of your abdomen with these rotations, moving from right to left.

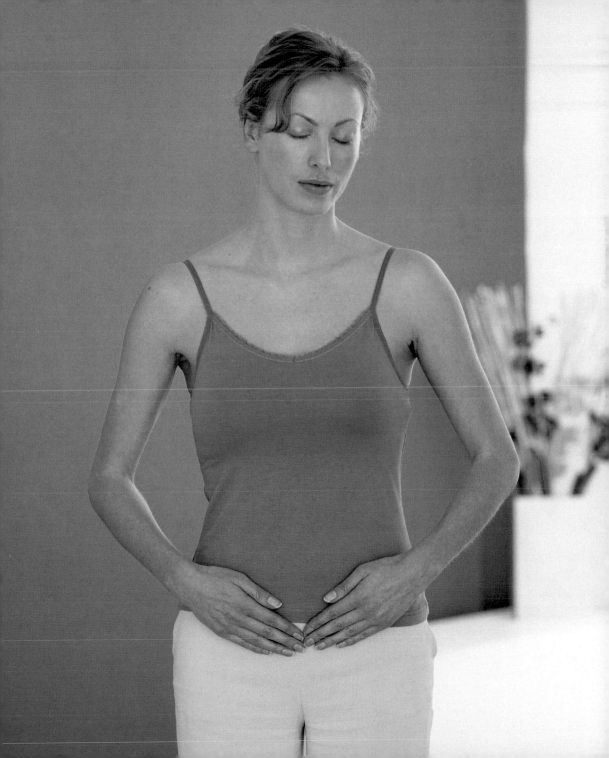

Arm swinging

If after working for hours your arms and shoulders ache, your brain refuses to cooperate, and your legs feel as if they've collapsed into your feet, you can revive yourself with a simple meditation and swinging routine. You may be surprised how little time it takes to rejuvenate with this routine.

Arm swinging is one of the traditional warm-up exercises that therapists use before starting work for the day. It warms up the muscles, relaxes the mind, and clears the energy channels, which is why it is useful as a limbering-up exercise before massage.

1. Stand with your feet about shoulder width apart and allow the weight of your head, neck, and shoulders to slide down your arms and out through your hands. Close your eyes if you wish, and feel all of the stress and tension in your upper body dripping from your fingertips down into the earth.
2. Slowly, pivoting your body around your waist, start to swing your arms. Allow them to move freely from your shoulders (see right).
3. Swing as far left as you can. Then, without breaking the rhythm, swing to the right as far as you can. Allow your hands to flop at the ends of your wrists. Keep the whole movement loose and free-flowing. Swing back and forth. Forget time. Forget everything but the feeling of dead weights at the end of your arms, slapping against your body when they land. Swing back and forth. Keep the rhythm slow and even. Breathe with the rhythm. Inhale and swing one way. Exhale and swing the other way. Keep your eyes closed and allow the swing to become automatic, just allow it to simply happen.

4. Breathe in. Swing, visualize a light coming into the top of your head, flowing down to your waist.
5. Breathe out. Swing, see this light moving down and out of your feet, carrying all your tiredness with it. See it moving deep into the earth. Keep this pumping action going at a slow, steady pace. If outside problems start to intrude, just observe them, watch them flow past your mind as if on a TV screen. They are not part of you at this moment. Let them go. Feel yourself within a great pillar of light, steadily filling

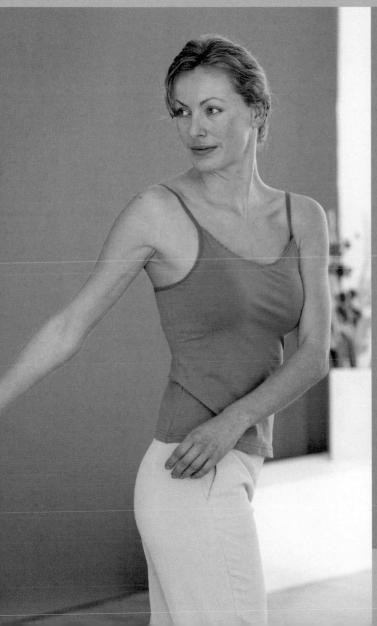

you up with energy.
6. Breathe in, feel your head filling with light.
7. Breathe out, feel the light flowing down your body, energizing and renewing your whole being.
On the in breath, slowly draw more and more energy into your body and mind. On the out breath, feel every last drop of tiredness leaving your body.
8. Feel the energy build with every breath, every swing. Remember to forget. See only yourself within this pillar of light. Physically connect with the light. If you feel your pace increasing slowly bring it back to a steady, comfortable swing. Be aware of the gentle slap of your hands against your body. Continue for as long as you wish. When you are ready, allow your hands to drop naturally by your sides. Take a few deep breaths and come back to full awareness.

Clearing your head

Heavy headaches, poor concentration, and eye strain often occur in the mid-afternoon, especially if you have spent hours working at a computer. Poor posture, shallow breathing, telephones, glaring computer screens, and electrical equipment that produces a build-up of static negativity around us cause a variety of minor health problems every day. To combat these it is worthwhile taking a few moments now and again to move stiff muscles, re-oxygenate the brain and body, and rest tired eyes. It can also be helpful to keep a quartz crystal by your computer to help absorb static and to rebalance the surrounding energy.

If you can, move away from your computer or, better still, try to take a brisk walk outside of the building to get some air that has not been fed through an air-conditioning system, if only for a couple of minutes.

HEADACHE AND EYE STRAIN

1. Taking both hands, reach as far as you can behind your head and down your back. Then strongly massage into your upper back on either side of your spine for about a minute.
2. Move your hands up to your neck and repeat as strongly as you can. The points to use are the two B10 on the back of the neck.
3. Hook your thumbs into the hollows either side of your neck just as it joins your head. Press in an upward direction while leaning your head back against your thumbs. Hold this position for as long as possible – for at least 30 seconds.
4. Slide all four fingers of both hands to the back of your neck at the base of your skull and press inward and upward with your fingertips. Lean back into this and hold for 30 seconds. This covers GB20 and GV16.
5. Place the heels of your hands either side of the back of your head, level with your crown, spacing your hands

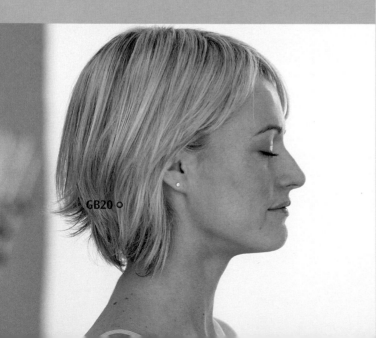

GB20 ○

so that you can just interlock your fingers over the top of your head. Now squeeze strongly with the heels of your hands in an upward direction. Hold for about 30 seconds. Release, move your hands midway toward the temples and repeat the squeeze. Move again so that the heels of your hands are against your temples and squeeze and hold again.

6. Place the palms of your hands over your eyes and relax into this position for three or four minutes. Press with your thumbs into the inner corners of your eyebrows, B2, for 30 seconds. Another good point is GV24.5 at the bridge of your nose between your eyes.

CONCENTRATION LOSS

1. Hold point GV26, just under your nose and above your two front teeth, and GB20, which you can find by running your fingers up either side of your head, just behind your ears, till they meet on the top of your head. Hold these points at the same time, with a firm pressure, while taking deep breaths. Visualize your breath moving down to your abdomen and back up through the top of your head. Do this for ten breaths.

2. Relax and repeat twice , taking breaks between each count of ten so that you do not cause dizziness.

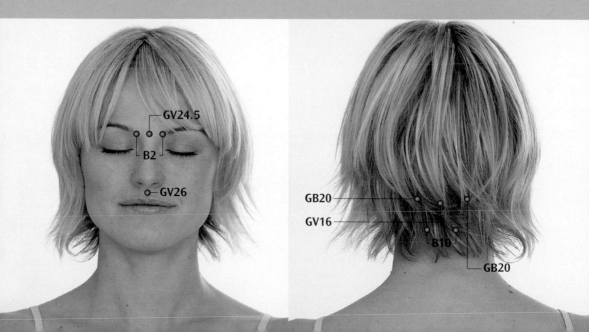

GV24.5

B2

GV26

GB20

GV16

B10

GB20

CHAPTER FIVE

Relaxing with head massage

It's the end of the day. You're home, warm, comfortable, and at peace? No? More often than not you'll have hot, swollen feet, an aching lower back, a muzzy head, a stiff neck, and more. This is because our bodies take quite a lot of punishment during an average day, causing us to feel less than well.

True relaxation can allow our bodies and minds to refresh themselves. When you arrive home it is worth taking time to make a conscious effort to break the connection with the day and its problems.

Lie flat on your back with your feet higher than your head for 20–30 minutes to enable the discs in your spine to re-inflate.

While you are lying there you can also help your head and body by palming. Place your hands on top of your head and feel their warmth. Observe this warmth, feel it penetrating your scalp and your brain. Breathe slowly and deeply. Feel your breath drawing the heat into your head. Take about three to five minutes in this position.

Move your hands to your face. Hold your palms lightly over your eyes and again feel the warmth of your hands. Relax all the tiny muscles around your eyes. Allow your face to dissolve. Breathe the warmth into your face.

After three to five minutes move your hands to your ears and feel the warmth in your ears. Allow your jaw to loosen. Feel your breath filling your whole head.

Move one hand over your heart and place the other over the tanden (lower abdomen). Deepen your breathing. Feel the in-breath moving down through your body to the tanden and the out-breath rising up through your body to your heart. Feel the warmth from your hands filling your whole body while you breathe. Try to keep this cycle going for the rest of the time you are lying down.

Head massage: setting the scene

Regular head massage not only benefits you by relaxing and loosening your shoulders, neck, and head but it also has a cumulative effect on your mental and emotional state. It can fire up your creativity. If you are struggling with a problem try this simple way of finding a solution. Condense the problem to a concise sentence. Repeat this to yourself three times, just before you have a head massage. Then forget it. Relax, enjoy your massage and by the time you have finished you will find that ideas will be pouring into your head. Don't try to make anything happen, just allow the process to run.

The techniques in this chapter have been taken from Indian head massage, Shiatsu, holistic massage, and others. They are gentle, releasing treatments, which are great for headache, stuffiness, stiff neck and shoulders, and have many other benefits. There are many pressure points within your face and head that connect with the whole of your being. These can be stimulated by stroking or toning, or if excess energy is the problem, as in the case of an inability to concentrate or focus, they can disperse this excess and calm your mind. Head massage also affects the pulsing rhythms of the cerebrospinal fluid which transmits healing around the body. This fluid runs up and down the spine and around the brain at a regular twelve cycles per minute carrying messages about the health and well-being of your whole system from the body to the brain and back again.

A COOL HEAD
In a calm, relaxed frame of mind tensions within your body will dissolve. Head massage is a wonderful way to achieve this state.

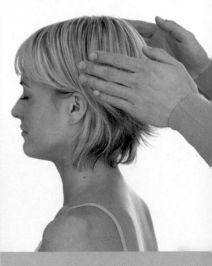

Back massage: heel of hand rotations

Every time your brain works fast, even if you are just watching an exciting film, the muscles in your back tense for action. In the average day this tension can build up to become an almost permanent state. Massaging strongly into the back muscles encourages these muscles to release this tension. Working with one arm supporting your partner allows them to feel safe and comfortable, allowing their mind as well as their body to relax and let go.

NOTES AND SUGGESTIONS
The pressure you use should be quite strong, but should not cause any pain.

1. Move to your partner's side so that you can provide support with your arm across the chest.
2. Place the heel of your other hand about two finger widths away from the far side of the spine, at shoulder level (see left).
3. Now lean strongly into the back as you rotate for a count of five with the heel of your hand on the spot.
4. Move about three finger widths out toward the shoulder and repeat the movement.
5. Do this until you reach the shoulder, then come back to the centre. Move your hand about a palm's width down the back and repeat the rotations across to the side.
6. Cover the side with rotations, then change sides so that you can work on the rest of the back.

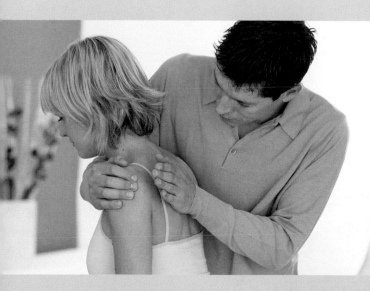

Shoulder/arm pinch

This massage is very good for loosening up the back of your neck and the large muscles of your shoulders and your upper arms, which take most of the strain when you are putting in long hours at a computer.

1. *Stand behind your partner and grasp the shoulders, either side of the neck. By pushing down with the heel of your hand and pulling with your fingers, pinch (don't nip) the flesh of the shoulders in a forward, rolling motion (01). The heels of your hands should slide toward your fingertips.*
2. *Move your hands about a palm's width out across the shoulders and repeat. You are now moving into a bonier area which could be painful, so be guided by how your partner feels about this.*
3. *Do the same movements down the arms to the hands, or as far as you can comfortably reach (02). If you can't do both shoulders and arms together, just do them one at a time, or substitute a wringing action for the pinch, which will also move the fibres of the muscles.*

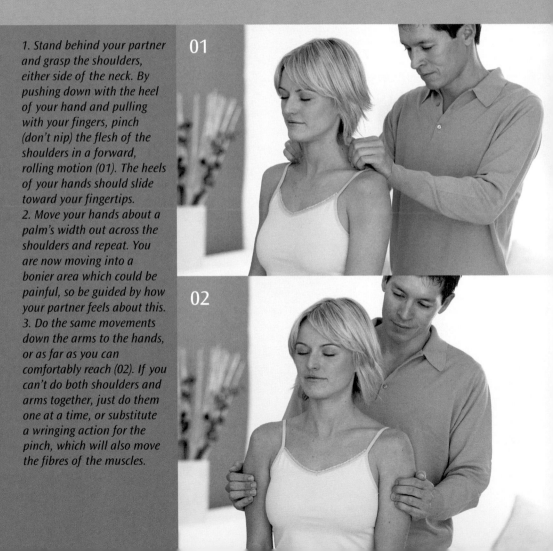

01

02

Elbow rotations

This intensive massage is very good for releasing stiff necks and shoulders, improving the flexibility of the neck so that you can turn to look behind you more easily, which is particularly useful when driving a car.

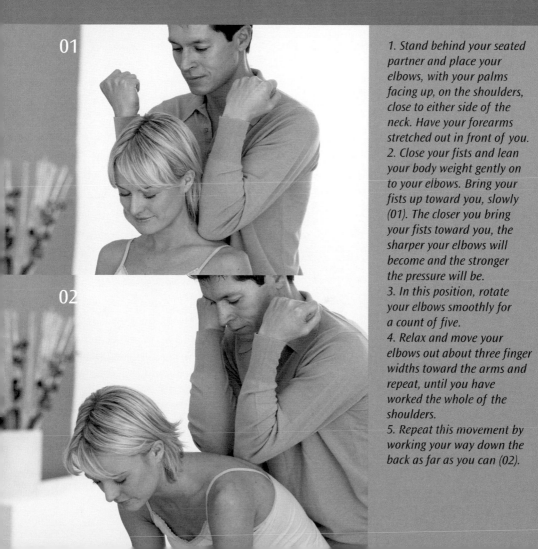

1. Stand behind your seated partner and place your elbows, with your palms facing up, on the shoulders, close to either side of the neck. Have your forearms stretched out in front of you.
2. Close your fists and lean your body weight gently on to your elbows. Bring your fists up toward you, slowly (01). The closer you bring your fists toward you, the sharper your elbows will become and the stronger the pressure will be.
3. In this position, rotate your elbows smoothly for a count of five.
4. Relax and move your elbows out about three finger widths toward the arms and repeat, until you have worked the whole of the shoulders.
5. Repeat this movement by working your way down the back as far as you can (02).

Neck workout and still points

Many headaches, eye strain, and facial aches start around the neck area. This massage not only releases your immediate pains and stiffness, it can also, if used regularly, greatly reduce the effects of migraine, realign your head/neck balance, so easing any long held postural problems, and it can also help to alleviate tension-related tinnitus. The still points (GB20) are very useful for draining a cold. If you feel sniffly, headachy, or just fuzzy, you can massage by rotating with your finger and thumb on these points for a few moments every half hour or so. Your cold should rapidly work its way out of your system. You can use this technique as a self-treatment.

CAUTION
■ *Do not use this massage on anyone with a medical neck condition.*

1. Still standing behind your partner, hold the forehead so that the head can drop forward slightly. With four fingers of the other hand, and starting about a finger's width from the spine, with your fingers running down the length of the vertebrae of the neck, gently rotate your fingers for a count of ten. This movement should be slow and very flowing. Repeat the movement two or three times, working your fingers out away from the spine in a circular spiral.
2. Change hands and repeat on the other side of the neck.
3. When you have completed both sides, place your thumb and first finger on either side of the spine, close to the head, in the dimply areas where the vertebrae meet the skull (see left). Press strongly in an upward direction into these still points for a count of five, then relax.

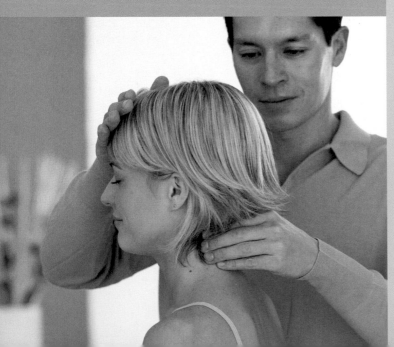

Head scratching/ Hair pulling

Scratching is a very enlivening technique which helps to clear the mind.

Hair pulling can be used in conjunction with rotations (see p.86) or pressure (see p.87), to ease headaches, as it moves any stagnant and blocked energy in the head. It works in the opposite way to rotations by pulling the scalp away from the skull. It helps to release pressure imbalances in your head. It also helps to strengthen your hair roots and can regulate the flow of oils in your hair, easing problems of excessive grease or dryness in the hair and scalp. You can use hair pulling as a self-treatment.

NOTES AND SUGGESTIONS

Keeping your fingernails in line while scratching will ensure that you do not snag the scalp.

HEAD SCRATCHING
You can do this with both hands or just one, with the other supporting your partner's forehead. Hold your hand(s) with the fingers curled so that your fingernails are in line with each other and scratch with a rapid, loose sideways action all over the head.

HAIR PULLING
1. Starting with both hands at the back of your partner's head, run your hands up into the hair with your fingers spread open until you have a handful.
2. Close your fingers on the hair and, keeping a firm hold on the hair, pull your hands away from your partner's head in a perpendicular direction, allowing the hair to slide through your fingers (see left). Do this until you have covered the whole head.

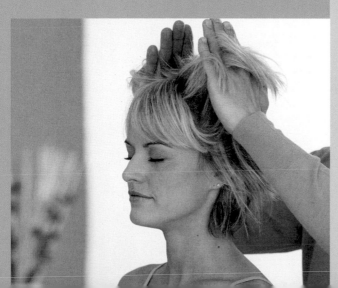

Hair stroking/ combing, rotations

Hair stroking or combing is a gentle, calming technique and is one of the few head massage strokes that can safely be used for cancer sufferers, the very young, the elderly, and those suffering from bone diseases. It releases stress and tension, gently stimulates the hair and scalp, eases depression, and can help in cases of insomnia and hyperactivity.

Rotations disperse any excess energy within the meridians of the head. You can use both techniques as self-treatment.

NOTES AND SUGGESTIONS

If your partner has long hair you may have to work in stages. If the hair is very short, open your fingers wide and, with a little pressure at the fingertips, start at the nape of the neck, following the same path as before.

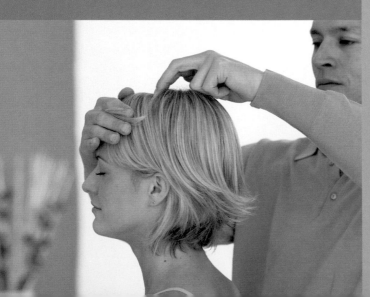

STROKING/COMBING

1. Still standing behind your partner, run both hands up into their hair.
2. Work with open fingers from the back of the neck to the forehead.
3. When you reach the hairline, comb your fingers through the hair, bringing your hands toward you. Then move your fingers up through the hair from the sides, starting just above the ears, up to the top of the head (see below left). Comb back through to the ears.

ROTATIONS

1. Hold your partner's forehead with one hand so that they can bend forward slightly.
2. With two fingers of your other hand, start at the centre of the hairline, working in small rotations back to the nape of the neck.
3. Return to the front of the head to a position two finger widths to the side of your first line. Continue along a line parallel to the first. Repeat, moving two finger widths to the side for each new line, until you reach the ear. Repeat on the other side of the head.

Head shake, pressure

'Head shake' loosens the scalp and stimulates a good blood and nutrient flow to the roots of the hair. It also strengthens the root system which can help in cases of hair loss. As you get used to this technique you can work more vigorously. Head shake is very effective as a self-treatment.

Pressure is a very still technique, useful for toning any low energy areas in the meridians in the head, which can help your whole body and mind to achieve good health and well-being. In therapies such as Shiatsu, calming techniques like these are the opposite of the more vigorous, rotating moves. They help to maintain the overall balance and energy flow within the meridians by allowing them to absorb healing energy. On a physical level pressure can help to stabilize any imbalances within the flow of the fluids around the brain and release pain and tension in stressed muscles. You can use this technique as a self-treatment.

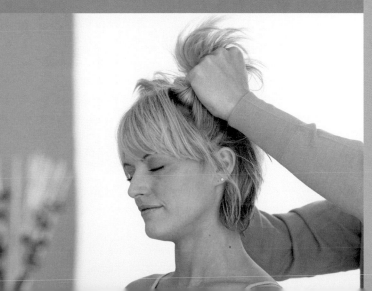

HEAD SHAKE

Run both hands into the hair and over the top of the head. When you have collected a handful, hold firmly and lightly shake the scalp back and forth (see below left). Don't pull hard, just enough to move the scalp.

PRESSURE

1. Hold your partner's forehead with one hand. With two fingers of your other hand, start at the centre of the hairline and exert a firm pressure for a count of ten.
2. Release and move about two finger widths back and repeat the pressure. Continue until you reach the base of the neck and finish the line by pressing upward into the base of the skull.
3. Go back to the hairline and move two finger widths to one side. You are following the same lines as in rotations. Now repeat the pressure along parallel lines until you reach the ear.
4. Comb your fingers through the hair and slowly allow your partner to take the weight of the head as you change hands and repeat the whole technique over the other side of the head.

Tapping, hacking

Light tapping produces a counterbalancing reaction within the whole head. It sends energizing ripples through the skull and brain, which wakes up all of the cells. If your head starts to feel sluggish during the day, a light, vigorous tapping on your own head can really get you going again. It can reduce the pain of headache caused by air conditioning or computer work, loosen up your neck and shoulders, and free your arms from the stiffness of immobility.

Hacking is a stronger massage technique than tapping, using the full weight of the hands and lower arms. Hacking works at a deeper level which frees up tension in the lower tissues within the muscles.

TAPPING
This can be done with both hands, but if your partner is very relaxed, support the head with one hand and work with the other.

TWO-HAND TAPPING
Starting at the hairline, use all fingers of both hands to tap back to the base of the neck, across the shoulders, and down the upper arms (01). Repeat two or three times, varying the line to cover the whole head, but always sweeping across the shoulders.

SINGLE-HAND TAPPING
Support the head with one hand and use the other to tap over the other side of the head and out along the shoulder two or three times. Repeat on the other side.

HACKING
Work with both hands, rapidly bouncing your hands off the head (02). Cover the whole of the head, neck, shoulders, and down over the upper back. This should be a whipping action.

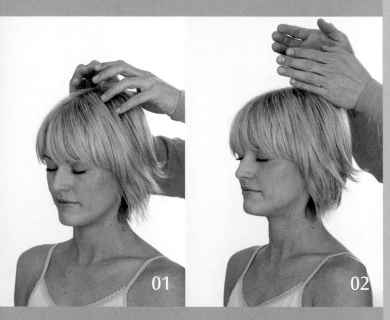

01

02

Ear massage

There are over two hundred acupuncture points within the ears which acupuncturists use to reach every part of your body. These can also be stimulated by pressure to help tone, stimulate, detox, and de-stress your whole being.

NOTES AND SUGGESTIONS
The ears will probably feel very hot when you have finished this massage.

1. Take hold of both of your partner's ears at the top, close to the head, between your finger and thumb.
2. Rub firmly while moving your grasp down around the outer edge of the ears to the lobes (01).
3. When you reach the lobes, pull down for a count of ten (02). Return to the tops and move down one finger width into the shells of the ears (03).
4. Repeat in a circular direction, following the shape of the ear. Massage firmly into all the nooks and crannies. When you have completed this, hold your hands over the ears for several moments.

Face stroking

This movement tones and conditions all of your facial muscles, encouraging them to fight against the forces of gravity. You will actually feel your face expanding as the tension dissolves away and wrinkles ease out.

1. Allow your partner to rest their head against you.
2. With both hands meeting under the chin, lightly stroke in an upward and outward direction (see right). Move your hands to meet under the nose and stroke again. Move your hands so that they meet on the nose and, avoiding the eyes, stroke upward and outward once more. Place your hands so that they meet on the forehead and stroke upward and outward again. Repeat this three or four times.

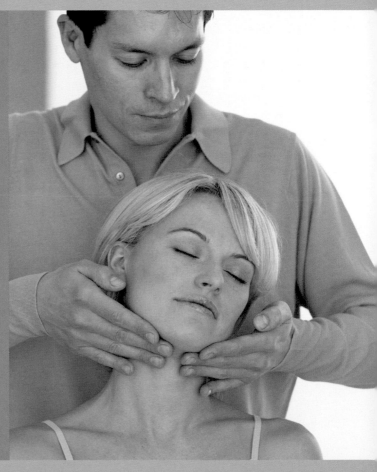

Muscle resistance

This not only wakes up your face and head but is also very good for strengthening the facial muscles and reducing wrinkle formation. It also helps with eye strain, sinus problems, and head and facial tension.

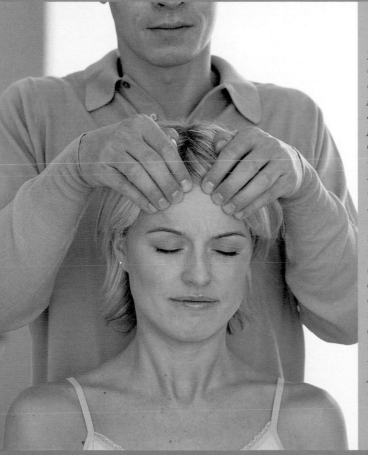

1. Place all of the fingertips of both hands in the centre of your partner's forehead (see left). Ask them to tense the muscles under your fingertips for a count of 10, then release.

2. Move your fingertips two finger widths apart so that you are working toward the temples and working both sides of the face at the same time. Tense and release.

3. Move your fingers two finger widths again and repeat. Do this until you reach the temples. Move your fingers to meet in the middle of the nose and tense and release, even over the eyes, until you reach the ears. Move down again to cover the area from the nose to the chin, tense and release.

4. Hold the sides of the face for a few moments before breaking the contact.

CHAPTER SIX

The whole works

The end of a day – whether it has been busy, stressful,
or just plain fun, is a time when you can relax, fall into
a wonderful soothing bath, and then enjoy an evening
just for the two of you. An hour or so of unwinding
massage provides healing, rejuvenating bliss – the
power of touch at its most potent.

Techniques taken from Shiatsu, holistic massage, Tantric massage, head massage, and other gentle, soothing routines can release all the tensions and stresses at the root of many of today's health problems. These techniques do not rely on strong manipulation, but on persuasion, relaxation, and release. Every cell in the body communicates with every other and if one part of the body feels under attack, this gives rise to tension, which can transmit itself to every part of our being. However, the deep, gentle techniques of holistic therapies will make us confident that there will be no sudden surprises and so will more readily submit to releasing stress.

The fascia, a fibrous connective tissue that runs through our bodies, touching and communicating with every living part, is very sensitive to stress. In fact, prolonged stress can produce solid knots and areas of almost unbreakable tension within this fascia, triggering deep-seated illness in organs such as the heart, lungs, and intestines. The strength of the fascia can vary from a fine web to strong diaphragms. If the membrane around your joints is under prolonged tension, it can cause misalignment. Regular deep relaxation, of which massage is a major part, can do much to relieve this imbalance.

Starting with a meditation that will connect you and your partner and release the pull of the outside world, then moving on to work with the yang protector areas of the body and, finally, with the more sensitive yin areas, this routine will allow body, mind, and spirit to completely renew and refresh themselves at the deepest level.

Creating the atmosphere

Prepare a cosy space in which to perform your massage. As the floor is the working area for this massage, ensure that you have enough room to allow your partner to lie full length in comfort, and to enable you to move freely without feeling cramped.

Place a couple of duvets or folded blankets on the floor, so that you have enough padding all around your partner to kneel or sit on. Have two or three small pillows or cushions to place under the head and shoulders when needed and a sheet or light blanket to cover your partner in the closing stages.

Play your favourite soft music to lead you through the massage unless you would prefer silence.

Use a light, subtle fragrance of your favourite oil in a carrier oil such as grapeseed on your hands, as this can help you both to move into a healing, meditative state. Oil burners are also useful, but take care with the strength of the fragrance.

If it is daylight outside draw the curtains. If you are not using oils in a burner or on your hands, then scented candles can provide aroma and soft lighting.

Good ventilation and an even, warm temperature are important. Sudden gusts of hot air from a fan heater can be distracting, even on a cool night, while a cool breeze in a hot room can be very pleasurable.

While you are setting up your room try to slow your breathing. Allow your movements to flow rhythmically. See this as a ritual for communication between you, your partner, and the universe.

Now try the meditation on pp.96–7 to synchronize your breathing and clear your energy flow.

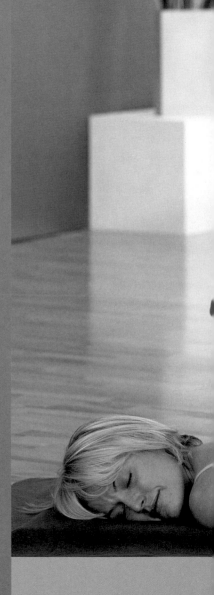

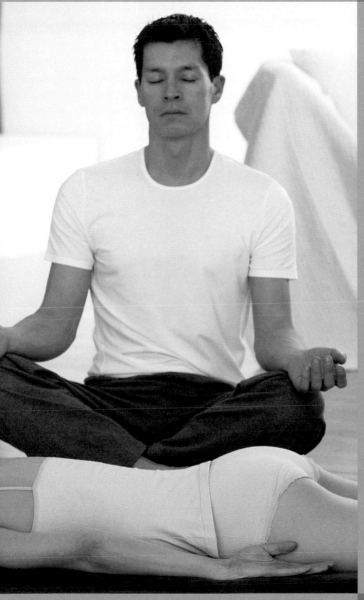

CHOOSING YOUR OILS

You can blend your own mixture of oils if you prefer. For a deep, woody scent you could use a few drops of frankincense with sandalwood. For a soft, floral aroma blend a few drops of geranium with chamomile. For a fresh, fruity scent use a few drops of lemongrass with basil. Lemongrass can also be used with the woody oils to lighten their scent. Frankincense can be added to the floral or citrus oils to deepen their perfume. But don't use too many oils in a mixture or they will fight each other.

Amber meditation

This meditation will help to clear your energies and those of the room. Amber is a fossilized plant resin. It is considered very healing and acts by absorbing negative energy and emitting positive energy. It is a calming, soothing, and relaxing stone which your partner may like to hold during the massage. Alternatively, place a few amber crystals around the room to help rebalance any negativity released during the treatment.

NOTES AND SUGGESTIONS

Work on a well-padded floor, using a couple of duvets or folded blankets.

For the massage, have your partner lie face down, forehead supported, so that the head and neck are straight and the arms are down by the sides.

If you find that your hands are feeling heavy, buzzy, or as if they are cloaked in cotton wool, give them a hard shake.

Visualize the static leaving your hands and disappearing into the earth. This will disperse any dense energy that you may have gathered while you were working.

1. Sit a relaxed arm's length opposite your partner. Gaze into each other's eyes for a few moments to see into each other's hearts.
2. Place your dominant hand on your partner's heart, placing your free hand over their hand that is on your heart (see right). Synchronize your breathing.
3. Close your eyes and imagine a warm amber mist filling the room. Allow the mist to move over your skin, sliding like a breeze.
4. Put your awareness into this feeling, allowing it to touch every part of you.
5. Feel the mist circling and swirling around the room, allowing your awareness to be carried with it. If thoughts from the day intrude, observe and let go.
6. Feel the mist moving under your skin, slipping just under the surface, moving deeper within you.
7. Feel the mist circling between the two of you, running from your hand to your partner's heart and

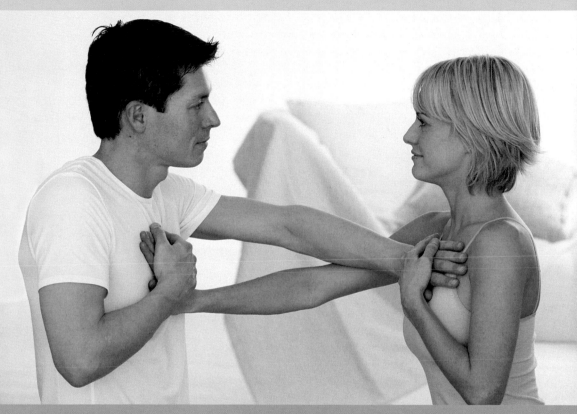

back from their hand to your heart. Allow this mist to circle for a few moments to build the connection between you.
8. Feel the circle growing out from you into the room, filling the room. Allow this circle to flow for a few moments.
9. Feel golden sparks shooting throughout the circle, energizing and cleansing the whole room.
10. Now slowly allow the mist to spiral down into the earth, taking with it any negativity and worries of the day, leaving behind a soothing, calm atmosphere.
11. Slowly have your partner lie face down and take position for your first massage move.

Tiger's claw

The full sequence of this massage moves energy at a very deep cellular level.

NOTES AND SUGGESTIONS
Work with both hands at the same time, following the rising yang and descending yin energy flow. Stand at your partner's feet. Hold your hands in a claw shape, with strong fingers. The hands are strong, but the touch is light. Move in a continuous flow, lightly running over the whole body. If you are going to do the whole massage sequence below, end the tiger's claw at the head, before turning your partner over.

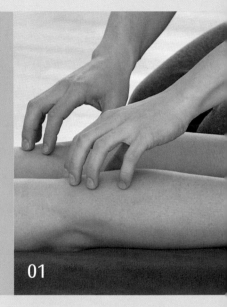

01

1. Start at the ankles and lightly stroke up the back of the calves to the knees (01). Move your hands out to the sides of the legs and stroke back down to the feet . Repeat three times, ending on the rising stroke, just behind the knees.
2. Continue the upward stroke over the buttocks to the hips (02). Move to the outside and downstroke to the knees. Repeat this line three times, ending on the upstroke level with the hips.
3. Continue the upstroke to

the shoulders (03). Move your hands out to the arms and stroke down the inner arms to the hands. Stroke up the outside of the arms and down the inside of the arms three times, ending on an upstroke at the shoulders.
4. Stroke both hands down your partner's sides to the hips. Move in toward the spine and stroke upward toward their shoulders (this follows the governing vessel). Repeat this three times, ending at the neck.
5. For the neck and head you

will need to close up the claw to the thumb and two or three fingers. Lightly stroke up the centre back of the neck to the crown of the head. Move your fingers out to each side of the head and stroke down to the base of the neck. Repeat three times.
6. If you are not going on to do the complete tiger's claw sequence, end here and go on to cat walking on back (see p.100). Otherwise, turn your partner over and continue.
7. Starting at the head,

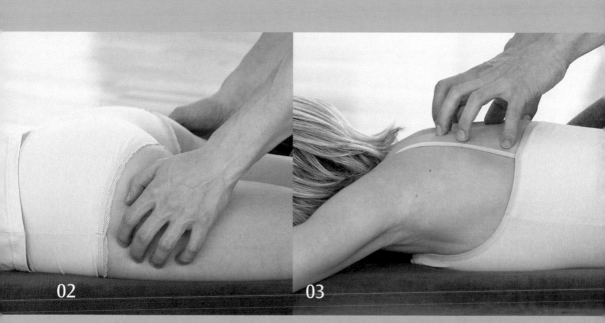

02

03

lightly stroke down the centre of the face and throat. At the base of the neck move your hands out to the sides and upstroke across the ears to the top of the head. Repeat three times, ending at the top of the sternum on a downstroke.
8. Move out to the arms and continue the downstroke over the outer sides of the arms, ending at the hands. Stroke up the inner arms to the shoulders. Repeat this three times, ending on an upstroke at the shoulders.

9. Move your hands back to the sternum. With one hand following the other down the centre of the body (this follows the conceptual vessel), move down until you reach the hara (lower abdomen). At the tanden, which is two finger widths below the navel, move your hands out to your partner's sides and stroke upward. Repeat three times, ending on a sideways stroke, stopping level with the tops of the thighs.
10. Stroke down the front

of the legs to the knees. Move to the outer side of the legs and stroke upward to the top of the legs. Repeat three times, ending on a downstroke at the knees.
11. Continue the downstroke to the feet. Do not work the soles as the light touch will tickle, destroying the relaxing effect. Move to the sides of the ankles and stroke up the sides of the legs to the knees. Repeat three times. End at the feet, holding them for a few moments.

Cat walking on back

This is a very deep treatment which works right down into the build-up of tight muscles that may not have fully relaxed for many years. You will feel a lot younger after only a few minutes of cat walking. Your stance will be more fluid and mobile and you will walk and move in a lighter way. This is a wonderful stretch for an aching lower back.

CAUTION
■ *Care must be taken in cases of clinical back problems or conditions.*

1. Position yourself above and facing your partner's head. Place your hands on the back, just below the neck and about two finger widths either side of the spine (01). Angle your fingers 45 degrees from the spine.
2. Kneel on one knee to improve your reach and balance. Slow your breathing to match your partner's, as

this will connect the two of you. Try to hold a feeling of warmth moving between the two of you throughout the whole treatment. Move slowly and try to feel your partner's response.
3. Walk hand over hand down the back, being careful not to put any weight on the spine (02). When you reach the base of the spinal area

hold that position for a moment (03). You should let your whole body weight rest on your hands.
4. Now slowly push yourself back, hand over hand, to your original position. Repeat at least three times.

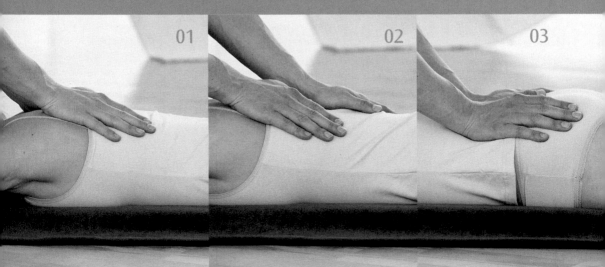

01 02 03

Side stretch

This technique is excellent for loosening up the entire back, releasing tension and pain.

NOTES AND SUGGESTIONS
If your partner has a very long back you may need to move two palm widths down after step 2 to reach the final stretch.

1. Move to your partner's right side. Starting on the shoulder area, place the heels of both hands about two finger widths away from the left side of the spine, with your fingers at right angles to the spine (01). Lean your weight slowly on to your hands and develop a push that will move the muscles of the upper back to stretch away from the spine. Hold for a count of ten.
2. Release and move your hands about two palm widths down the back. Put the heels of your hands about two finger widths away from the left side of the spine, fingers at right angles to the spine, and lean into the stretch, dropping your weight slowly on to your hands. Hold for a count of ten, then release.
3. Repeat, moving another two palm widths down the body. You should have one hand on the left hip, one on the waist (02). Angle the stretch at about 60 degrees to the spine, pushing out and down.
4. Move to the opposite side and repeat the sequence.

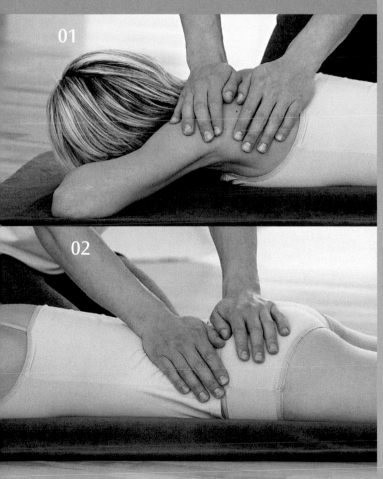

01

02

Cross stretching

This stretches all the muscles of the back in directions that move the muscle fibres over each other, helping to release toxin build-up within the muscles. It encourages a good flow of blood to all of your back muscles and frees up any locks in your spinal area.

CAUTION
Great care must be taken if your partner has clinical back problems.

1. Place your right hand on the right hip and your left hand on the left shoulder blade. Slowly drop your weight on to your hands in a crossways stretch. Hold for a count of three (01).
2. Release and change your hand positions so that your right hand is on the left hip and your left hand is on the right shoulder blade. Drop into the stretch and hold for a count of three (02).
3. Release. Leaving your right hand on the left hip, place your left hand under the right rib cage. Drop your weight into the stretch. Hold for a count of three (03).
4. Release, move your right hand over to the right hip and cross your left hand over to hold the left rib cage. Drop into the stretch. Hold for a count of three (04).
5. Release. Now cross your arms level with your partner's waist, placing your hands on their body, pointing away from each other, and pushing away from the spine in each case. Stretch, hold for a count of three (05), and release.

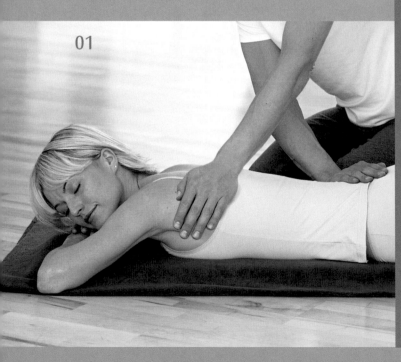

01

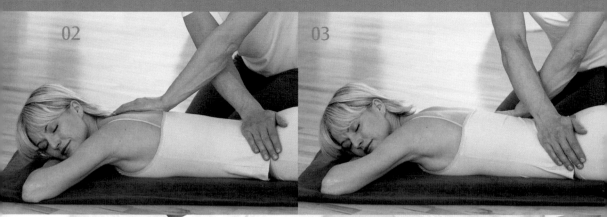

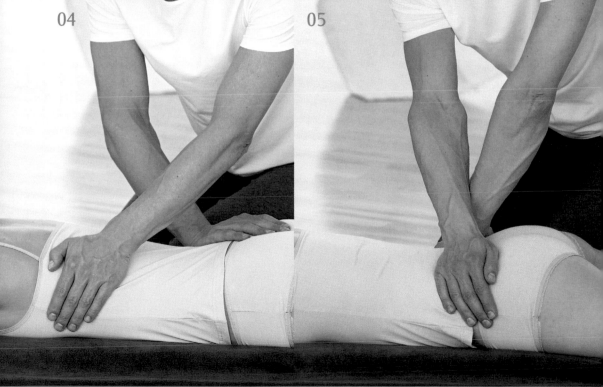

Back massage techniques

HACKING

You and your partner should breathe deeply during this movement to maximize the oxygenation of your bodies. Hold your hands loosely so that your fingers curl naturally. With swift, free-flowing wrists and hands, hack lightly over the whole back – this should be a whipping rather than a beating motion. It should be done with care, since, if performed too vigorously by untrained hands, it could hurt your wrists. Starting from one buttock move in a circular direction up the back, across the shoulders, down the other side of the back, and over the buttocks. Continue this movement for three to four circuits. Then rest. This is very energizing and enlivening for both of you (see also p.88).

BACK ROTATIONS

Hold your partner's shoulder with one hand, referred to as the listening hand. You don't need to pay too much attention to this hand, just be aware of any changes in your partner as you work with your other hand. With the fingers of your working hand, start about two finger widths away from the spine, at shoulder level, and move away from the spine and your listening hand. The pressure should be firm without being painful. Work your fingers in small rotations over a small area for a count of three to five (01, 02). Then move about three finger widths in the direction of your partner's side and repeat. Continue until you reach your partner's side, then come back to the spine. Drop your hand about a palm

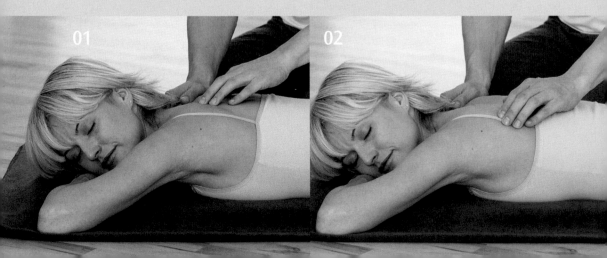

01

02

width down the back and start the rotations again. Cover that side of the back then move to the other side of the body, changing hands so that the listening hand and the working hand swap places, and cover the rest of the back with rotations. If the pressure is kept firm, this technique gives a deep soothing massage that will break down any long-held tension.

WORKING THE VERTEBRAE

Still holding your partner's shoulder with the listening hand, loosen the spine by working each vertebra. Use your thumb and three fingers of your working hand to grasp each vertebra in turn and move it in a circular motion for a count of three (03), starting at the base of the neck and working down to

the coccyx. This frees up the whole spine, making it mobile and supple.

TIGER'S CLAW

This is a short, figure-of-eight variation, for the back only. You can use one hand or both. If you are working with one hand, use your other to "listen". Start at the middle top of the back, holding your hand lightly in the shape of a claw, with strong fingers. Stroke in a figure of eight across your partner's upper back for seven circuits. Then, slide your hand down to mid back, without breaking the rhythm, and do another seven circuits (04). Move down again to the lower back and repeat the seven circuits.

If you want to work with both hands you will find details of the technique on pp.98–9.

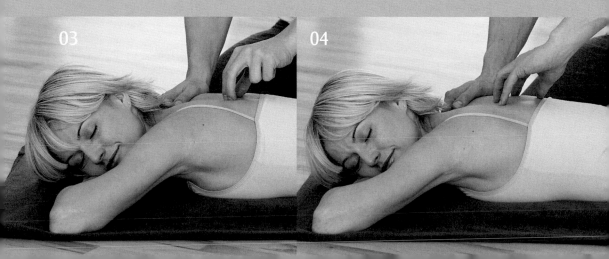

03

04

Palming down legs

This is a light massage which will encourage good
circulation of blood and lymph fluids within your legs.
It relaxes the large muscles in your legs, helping to
ease out back and leg pains caused by bad posture.
Massaging can be just as beneficial for the giver.
If you allow yourself to move freely and work to
your extreme, your balance and flexibility
will improve greatly.

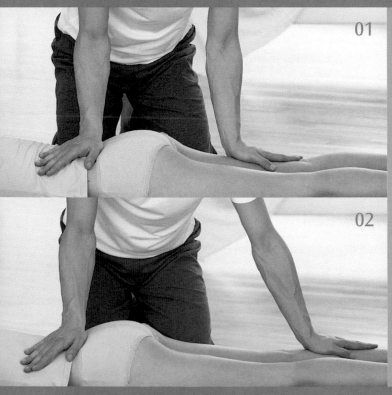

01

02

1. Place your listening hand
on the base of your partner's
spine and the other on the
top of the back of the thigh
nearest to you, with the heel
of your hand toward the
buttocks and the fingers
angled outward toward the
side of the legs (01).
2. Lean your weight fully on
to your working hand and
hold for a count of five.
Move a hand's length down
the leg and lean in again,
holding for a count of five.
3. Repeat all the way down
the leg until you reach the
foot (02), avoiding pressure
on the knees.
4. Repeat on the other leg.

Wringing out calves

This is a more vigorous massage which works strongly on the muscles of the calves. The movement is like that used when wringing out wet clothes, and it literally squeezes toxins out of the muscle fibres. It also works to dispel any stagnant blood that has pooled in the lower legs.

CAUTION
■ *This massage should not be attempted if your partner has varicose veins.*

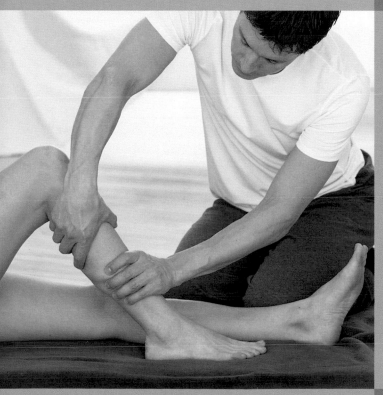

1. Hold one of your partner's calves with two hands and, starting just below the knee, wring out as you would a wet garment, moving down the leg to the foot (see left).
2. Repeat on the other leg.
3. End by sitting at your partner's feet and holding them for a few moments. Pick up the feet and support both of them over your lap. Now begin working the feet and ankles (see pp.108–9).

Rotating ankles

The load-bearing joints of your ankles take a huge amount of strain on even the most sedentary day. Imagine holding your own weight in your hands as you get out of bed in the morning. It would be quite an effort, yet that is the strain your ankles take every time you get up from a chair, climb stairs, or do anything that moves your weight from one foot to the other. To combat this strain, your ankle joint can, over time, sometimes hold a permanent tension. This can cause pain and stiffness and also trap waste cellular matter within the joint. Rotating your ankles in a way that is not load-bearing can help to free this stiffness, improving the overall mobility and strength of your ankle joints.

CAUTION

■ *Care must be taken if your partner has any damage to the joints.*

1. Hold one of your partner's ankles in one hand (01). Grasp the foot with the other hand and move it in a smooth circular rotation (02). Be careful not to cause any pain, but try to explore the full movement of the ankle. Work first in one direction, then the other.
2. Continue with the stretching (see p.109) and a massage (see p.110) before moving on to the other foot.

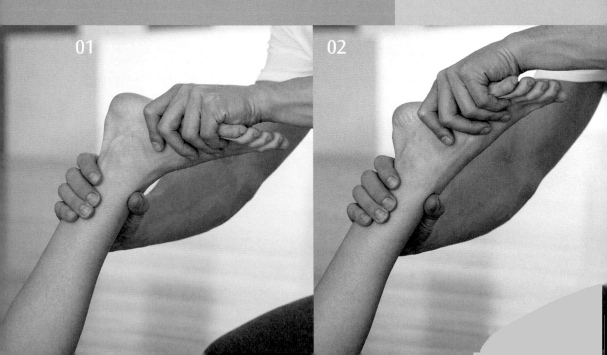

01

02

Stretching feet

As your ankle starts to stiffen, more strain is placed on other areas of your feet. This sequence will ease out any tense muscles and stretch the tendons of your ankle and foot. It will also free up any immobility in your toes, helping your balance and bringing a lighter, flowing quality to your gait. You'll walk taller and feel more energetic after this massage.

1. Hold your partner's ankle with one hand. Place the working hand over the heel and, lean into your hand with your forearm. Press it along the sole of the foot, stretching it as far as it will go, with the toes moving toward the knee (see left).
2. Change the position of your working hand and hold the top of the foot.
3. Now stretch the foot in the other direction, pointing the toes as far as they will go.
4. Finish this foot with rotations and toe pulling (see p.110) before repeating the whole sequence on the other foot.

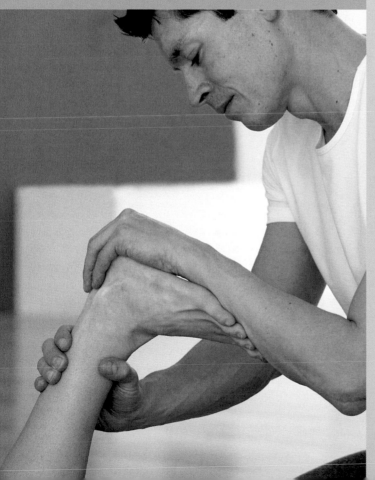

Rotations over the feet and toe pulling

This increases the flexibility of the feet and helps to move any toxin build-up. It also works many of the meridians of the body, such as the lung, large intestine, stomach, spleen, heart, small intestine, bladder, kidney, liver, and gall bladder, promoting overall good health and well-being.

NOTES AND SUGGESTIONS

This is a simple massage which you can also use as a self-treatment to relieve tired feet and help you get through the most trying day. As the old saying goes – "What goes on in your feet shows in your face."

1. Support your partner's foot by holding the top of the foot, with the sole facing you.
2. Starting at the heel and moving along the outer edge of the foot work your thumb quite firmly (light pressure tickles) in small circles for a count of five in each position (01). Move down the edge about two finger widths and repeat until you reach the little toe.
3. Grasp the little toe firmly and pull, holding the stretch for a count of three.
4. Go back to the heel, move one finger width in toward the inner side of the foot, and repeat the sequence.
5. Do this three more times until you have covered the whole foot and pulled each toe in turn (02).
6. Now repeat, this time doing the rotations with your fingers over the top of the foot and following four lines between the bones of the foot down toward the toes. Repeat the whole sequence from the ankle rotation (p.108) on the other foot.

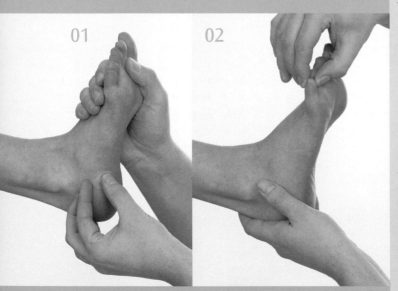

01

02

Finishing off

This closing sequence follows the rising yang and descending yin energies of the body, which helps to smooth out any remaining ripples of unbalanced energy in the back. It also pulls your energy away from your partner as they turn over for the front massage.

NOTES AND SUGGESTIONS
If your partner is very relaxed at this point and is close to sleep, closing the back with an energy sweep means that you can leave the massage here without your partner feeling only half done.

1. Using your whole hand, stroke up the back of the calves to the knees and down the sides of the legs to the feet three times (01).
2. On the third sweep continue up the back of the legs to the hips and then down to the knees three times (02).
3. Sweep up the back to the shoulders and down the sides to the base of the spine three times (03).
4. Ask your partner to turn over and continue.

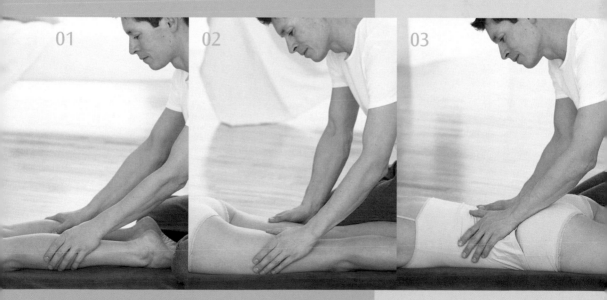

Knee swings

This is a lovely stretch for the lower spine. It gently moves apart the vertebrae of the mid and lower spine, releasing any long-held tension.

NOTES AND SUGGESTIONS
If your partner can't relax into the swing or feels insecure about you being able to carry their weight, you can simply lean back while holding their knees and stretch the spine without lifting the body from the floor. This way you will both gain confidence in each other's abilities and eventually you and your partner will be able to relax fully into this exercise.

CAUTION
■ *Great care must be taken if your partner has a clinical back problem.*

1. Stand with your legs apart, feet either side of your partner's knees. Pick up her knees (see right). If the legs remain tense, ask her to relax and allow her feet to drop to the floor.
2. Use your bent knees to support your elbows. Lean back to lift your partner's lower body off the floor.
3. Gently swing your partner from side to side about six to eight times.

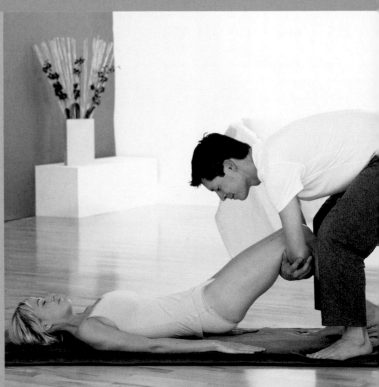

Knee stretches

This is a more strenuous stretch, which works deeply into the rotating action of the back. Your partner will feel wonderful after it.

NOTES AND SUGGESTIONS
You may find that your partner will resist this stretch as it is moving the body in an unusual way. If you feel them tensing ask them to make a deep inhalation and exhalation. You should be able to stretch a further 3–4 cm (1–1½ in) more and this will release their back. You may even find that their back crackles slightly as it frees up. But don't go so far as to cause pain.

1. Push your partner's knees up toward her chest, and hold for a count of five (01). To extend the stretch, lower the knees to the floor on one side (02), but do not allow her opposite shoulder to lift. If that happens, use one hand to hold down the knees and the other to hold down the shoulder. Hold for five.
2. Raise the knees to the centre and stretch to the other side.
3. Come back to centre. Slide your hands to grasp the ankles, shake them to loosen the whole body, and slowly lower the legs to the floor.

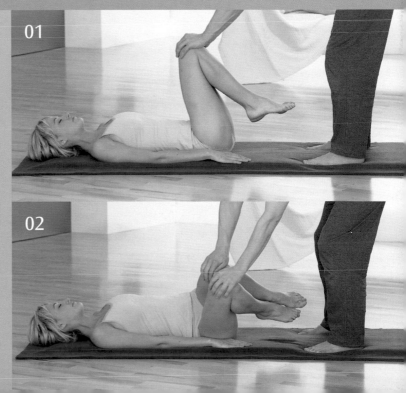

Arm stretching/wringing

Arm stretching uses the weight of your partner's body to gently release tension in their arms, shoulders, and upper back. By stretching the arms in this way you are assisting the flow of blood within the fibres of the muscles and easing those fibres over each other, allowing toxins and cellular debris to be dissolved by the blood and lymph fluids and carried away. The muscles themselves are also being stretched and released like an elastic band, which helps to relax the whole of the upper body.

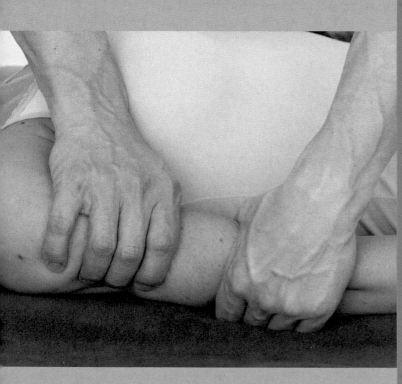

ARM STRETCHING

1. Stand behind your partner's head and take her hands.
2. Holding the wrists in both of your hands bend your knees and use them to support your elbows as you lean back and stretch your partner's upper spine (see p.112). Don't lift the body from the floor as the neck could twist uncomfortably. Just put their arms under tension and shake gently.
3. If you wish, from this position you could sit down on the floor, place your feet on your partner's shoulders, and stretch the arms by pulling with your hands and pushing with your feet. Don't push too hard, just enough to ease out any shoulder stiffness. Return your partner's arms to their sides.

ARM WRINGING

1. Sit by your partner's side and hold the opposite upper arm with both hands.
2. Work your way down the arm using a wringing motion (see left). Massage the hand, then work on the other arm.

Hand squeezing

This is a more intensive treatment for the hands, which works more strongly on the tissues to move any deep build-up of cellular debris and toxin deposits. This helps to free off any long-term stiffness in the muscles and joints, particularly in the hands and wrists. You will also cover many of the meridians that are found in the feet, giving a well-balanced treatment which will help to maintain good health. The squeezing can also be used as quick, effective, refreshing, and pain-relieving self-treatment.

1. Massage your partner's hand by squeezing it between your fingers and thumb as if making pastry, rubbing with your fingers on the back of the hand and with your thumbs over the palm (see left).
2. Work strongly from the heel of the hand to the fingertips, starting at the outer edge, up the little finger, and progressing over the hand toward the thumb.
3. Repeat the sequence of arm wringing and squeezing on the other hand.

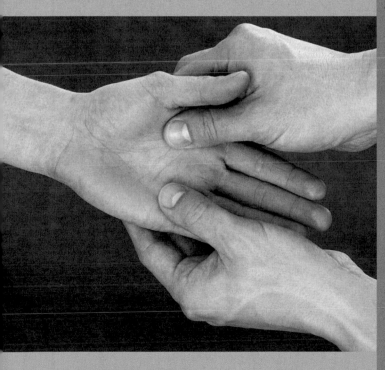

Abdomen: palm rolls

This is a particularly good treatment for anyone with digestive or elimination problems, as the palm rolls stimulate the organs within your abdominal area. Working from right to left encourages the flow of waste products through the intestines, the circulation of blood and other fluids through the kidneys and liver, and a healthy bowel action. Health problems such as irritable bowel syndrome (IBS) and Crohn's disease can be helped by the calming effect of palm rolls and the bowl (see p.117). Palm rolls also gently stimulate the meridians that pass through the abdominal area.

NOTES AND SUGGESTIONS
Releasing emotional problems can trigger a reaction that may last for a few days, but your partner will feel very much better and freer for this release.

1. Sit at your partner's right side, level with the abdomen. Place your hands on the abdomen, fingers closed (01). Hold for a moment to allow your partner to relax fully.
2. Lean your weight gently on to the heels of your hands (02). In a wavelike motion slowly roll your weight through your hands to the fingertips (03).
3. Lean back to return your weight to the starting position and repeat the wave seven to ten times. The rolling action should be smooth and flowing with medium pressure.

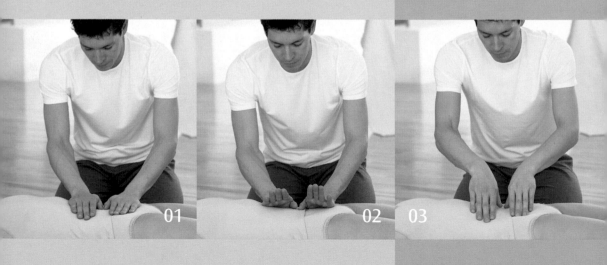

01

02

03

Abdomen: bowl

The bowl is very good for digestive and elimination problems. It is a gentler action than palm rolls and is very soothing and calming. It also stimulates the yin meridians which run from the head down through the body and into the feet. This gives a gentle workout for the conceptual/directing vessel, stomach, kidney, lung (through the lung extension), spleen, liver, and large intestine channels. It can help to stretch the fascia within the abdominal area. It is very calming and, as it also works the solar plexus and hara (lower abdomen) areas, it can help to release emotional problems.

NOTES AND SUGGESTIONS
As for palm rolls (see p.116).

1. In the same position as for the palm rolls, lift the inner sides of your hands so that they form a bowl shape (01).
2. Rock your weight in a circular motion so that it rolls clockwise around the rim of the bowl. Move with your whole body for seven to ten circuits.
3. When you have completed this, lightly hold your hands over the abdomen (02). Hold this position for a few moments. Observe your partner's breathing, slowly allowing their body to fall away from your hands.
4. Cover your partner with a sheet or light blanket and seat yourself at their head for the neck and shoulder workout and head massage.

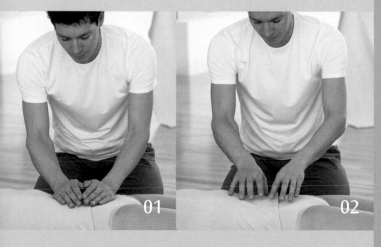

01   02

Neck and shoulder workout

Strong massage around your neck and shoulders
releases tension headaches, eye strain, facial pain, and
stiff muscles in your neck, shoulders, arms, and hands.

*1. Sit behind your partner,
place your hands above her
shoulders (01), and slide
them under the shoulders,
close to the spine.*
*2. Using your partner's body
weight to increase the
strength of the work, make
claws and, moving one hand
after the other in an upward
rolling action, work into the
shoulder area and neck for
a slow count of ten (02).*
*3. Place the inside edges of
your hands under the base
of your partner's neck, with
your forefingers touching the
neck and your little fingers
against the floor.*
*4. Working hand over hand,
pull strongly upward under
your partner's neck, from
base to top. Repeat this
action for a slow count of
ten, ending with one hand
supporting the base of
your partner's skull.*

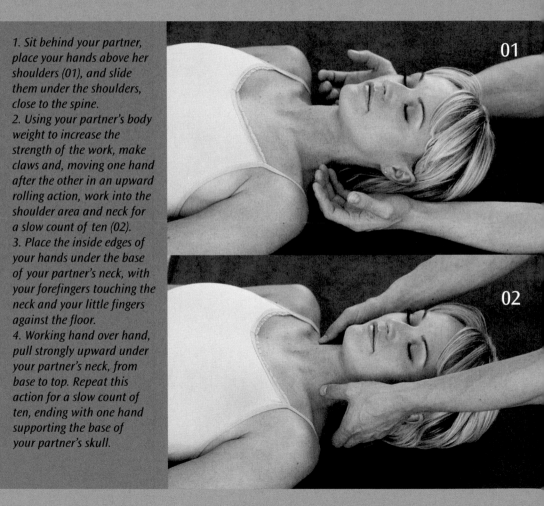

01

02

Head rotations, combing, stroking, pressure, hair pulling

These techniques are helpful for stress and headaches.

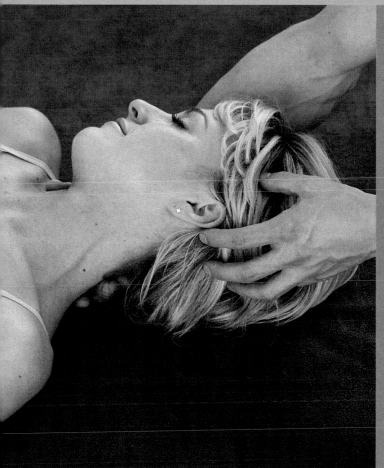

ROTATIONS

1. Tilt your partner's head to one side (see left). With the fingers of your free hand, starting at the base of your partner's skull, rotate upward toward the crown. The pressure should be firm without pulling or causing any pain.

2. When you reach the crown, move the head to face forward. Still supporting the head with one hand, continue the rotations right up to the hairline.

3. Using both hands, one each side of the head, and starting as far back as you can reach, work the rotations along the sides of the head until you reach the hairline.

COMBING AND STROKING

Comb your fingers upward and outward through the hair and stroke gently down over the hair. Repeat as many times as you wish.

PRESSURE

1. Support your partner's head with one hand and turn it to one side. With the fingers of the other hand, start at the base of the skull and exert a firm pressure for a count of three (01).

2. Move two finger widths up toward the crown and press in with your fingers for a count of three. Repeat until you reach the crown.

3. Turn the head to the front and continue with both hands along the sides of the head to the hairline, just in front of the ears.

4. Press both thumbs across the forehead, from the sides toward the centre (02).

5. When your thumbs meet, change direction. Work from the centre of the forehead to the crown (03). Bring your thumbs to the forehead and out two finger widths.

6. Work two lines parallel to the centre, toward the crown. Repeat two finger widths out again, to the outer edge of the head, before it curves down. Go over the whole head with more combing and stroking.

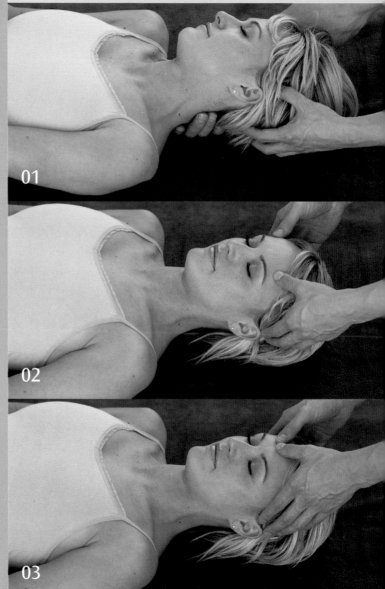

HAIR PULLING

1. Slide both of your hands, with open fingers, through the hair at the side of your partner's head until you have collected a good handful of hair.

2. Close up your fingers and pull outward in a direction perpendicular to the scalp (01). Repeat all over the head. This is a wonderful technique for relieving a headache.

3. Go over the whole head with combing and stroking (02). You can also follow this with any of the techniques you choose from the full head massage sequence (see pp.78–91).

4. Close the treatment by holding your partner's head for a few moments before slowly withdrawing your hands (03).

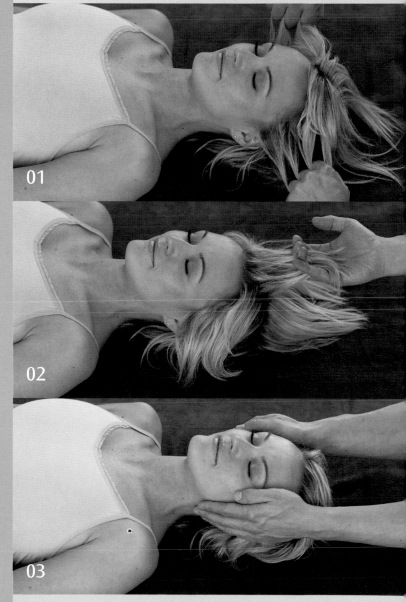

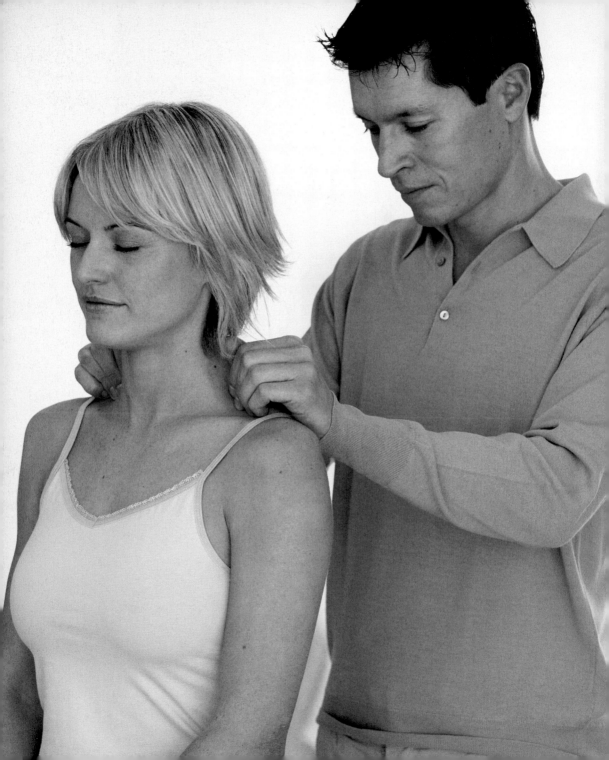

Further reading

Alexander, Jane
Five-Minute Healer
Gaia Books, 1999

Baker, Ian A.
The Tibetan Art of Healing
Thames and Hudson, 1997

Bentley, Eilean
Step-by-Step Head Massage
Gaia Books, 2000

Burmeister, Alice and
Monte, Tom
The Touch of Healing
(Jin Shin Jyutsu)
Bantam Books, 1997

Chaitow, Leon
Positional Release
Techniques
Churchill Livingstone, 1996

Chia, Mantak
Awaken Healing Energy
Through the Tao
Aurora Press,1983

Evans, Mark
Instant Stretches
Lorenz Books, 1996

Frantzis, B.K.
Opening the Energy Gates
of Your Body
North Atlantic Books, 1993

Gach, Michael Reed
Acupressure
Piatkus, 1990

Gillanders, Ann
BPG Reflexology
Gaia Books, 2002

Jarmey, Chris and
Mojay, Gabriel
Shiatsu – The Complete
Guide
Thorsons, 1991

Jarmey, Chris and
Tindall, John
Acupressure for Common
Ailments
Gaia Books, 1991

Lundberg, Paul
The Book of Shiatsu
Gaia Books, 1992

Masunaga, Shizut and
Ohashi, Wataru
Zen Shiatsu
Japan Publications, 1977

Melody
Love is in the Earth
Earth-Love Pub, 1995

Metzger, Wolfgang and
Zhou, Peifang
Tai Chi Chuan and Qigong
Sterling books, 1996

Rich, Penny
Practical Aromatherapy
Siena Books, 1996

Shen, Peijian
Massage for Pain Relief
Gaia Books, 1996

Szwillus, Marlisa
Mood Food
Gaia Books, 1999

Taylor, Kylea
The Breathwork Experience
Hanford Mead, 1994

Index

Acknowledgements

Author's acknowledgements

I would like to express my grateful thanks to all my relatives, friends, students, and teachers who have helped me in many ways to complete this book, in particular, Shiatsu Master Tutor Howard Malpas, who first introduced me to complementary therapies many years ago and has since, with his wife Elsa, been a great friend and teacher. I would also like to thank all at Gaia Books, Bridgewater Books, Mike Hemsley, and models Nikki and Adam, for all their help and hard work in producing this book.

Author details

Eilean Bentley is a member of the International Shiatsu Commission and E.A.R. (Acupuncture register). She is a master in Reiki, Seichim, and Karuna healing, and has studied Indian head massage and shamanic healing. She teaches privately and in adult and further education centres in and around London, and treats private clients as well as patients in the detox unit of an NHS hospital in the South of England. She is the author of *Step-by-Step Head Massage,* also published by Gaia Books.

Contraindications

Massage is a very safe therapy. However, sometimes you may have some reactions which can last for a few days. These are mainly of a detoxing nature, such as headaches and digestive or emotional upsets or problems.

Other cautions

Care is needed when treating the very young, the elderly, and those suffering from bone problems, epilepsy, clinical depression, cancer, low or high blood pressure, or who are pregnant. In these cases use only a very short, light massage.

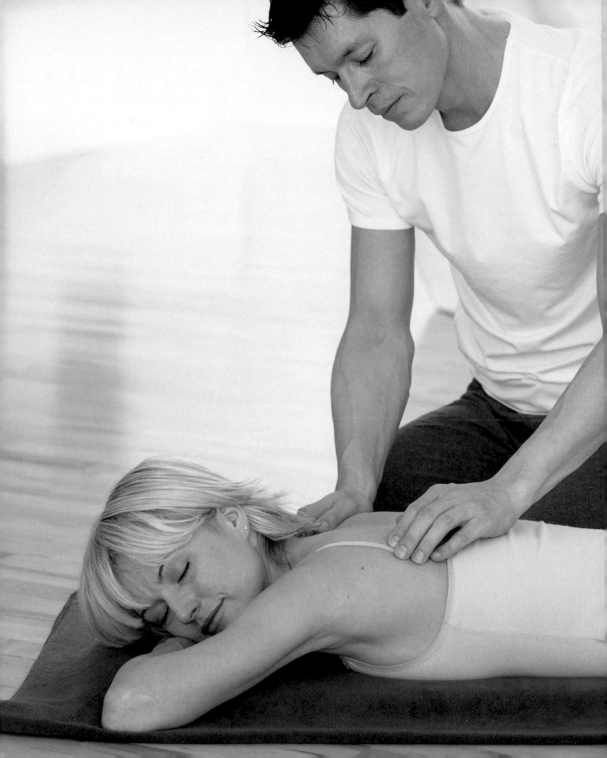